STRONG AND SEXY

INTERVIEWS WITH PERSONAL TRAINERS WERE DONE ORIGINALLY FOR AFTON BLADET, SOFI'S MODE. PT TIPS AND CERTAIN OTHER PORTIONS OF THE TEXT WERE PUBLISHED PREVIOUSLY IN SOFI'S MODE BUT HAVE BEEN REWORKED FOR THIS BOOK.

COPYRIGHT © 2012 BY SOFI FAHRMAN AND JULIA FORS AND NORSTEDTS, STOCKHOLM

ENGLISH TRANSLATION © 2015 BY SKYHORSE PUBLISHING

FIRST PUBLISHED BY NORSTEDTS, SWEDEN IN 2012 AS *BODYLICIOUS* BY SOFI FARHMAN AND JULIA FORS. PUBLISHED BY AGREEMENT WITH NORSTEDTS AGENCY.

EXPERT REVIEW FOR FITNESS PROGRAMS: SARA CLAESSON

HAIR AND MAKEUP: SARA ERIKSSON

DESIGN: FRIDA AXIÖ OF FRIDA STHLM. AB

COVER: FRIDA AXIÖ OF FRIDA STHLM. AB, PHOTO: JOHNNY WOHLIN

BODY PHOTOS: FREDRIK STREIFFERT, PP. 4, 6, 18, 19, 21, 76-81, 82, 83, 84, 89, 92, 95, 98, 100, 102-103, 104, 107, 108, 114, 115, 117, 118, 120, 123, 125, 126, 130, 131, 135, 141, 142, 151, 155, 157, 158-159

SUSANNE KINDT, PP. 8, 15, 16, 18, 22-74, 83, 84, 85, 86, 91, 116, 137, 140, 144, 150, 152-153, 154

SHUTTERSTOCK, P. 119; ANNA LUNDELL, P. 113; OTHERS FROM PRIVATE SOURCES

PRINTING: FÄLTH & HÄSSLER, VÄRNAMO

SKYHORSE EDITION EDITED BY AMY LI

SKYHORSE PUBLISHING BOOKS MAY BE PURCHASED IN BULK AT SPECIAL DISCOUNTS FOR SALES PROMOTION, CORPORATE GIFTS, FUND-RAISING, OR EDUCATIONAL PURPOSES. SPECIAL EDITIONS CAN ALSO BE CREATED TO SPECIFICATIONS. FOR DETAILS, CONTACT THE SPECIAL SALES DEPARTMENT, SKYHORSE PUBLISHING, 307 WEST 36TH STREET, 11TH FLOOR, NEW YORK, NY 10018 OR INFO@SKYHORSEPUBLISHING.COM.

SKYHORSE® AND SKYHORSE PUBLISHING® ARE REGISTERED TRADEMARKS OF SKYHORSE PUBLISHING, INC.®, A DELAWARE CORPORATION.

WWW.SKYHORSEPUBLISHING.COM

10 9 8 7 6 5 4 3 2 1

LIBRARY OF CONGRESS CATALOGING-IN-PUBLICATION DATA IS AVAILABLE ON FILE.

ISBN: 978-1-62914-411-5

EBOOK ISBN: 978-1-63220-137-9

PRINTED IN CHINA

SOFI FAHRMAN & JULIA FORS

STRONG AND SEXY

EXERCISE, FOOD, AND MOTIVATION FOR A HEALTHY BEACH-READY BODY

PHOTOS: SUSANNE KINDT AND FREDRIK STREIFFERT

Translated by Cory Klingsporn

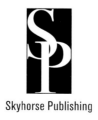

Skyhorse Publishing

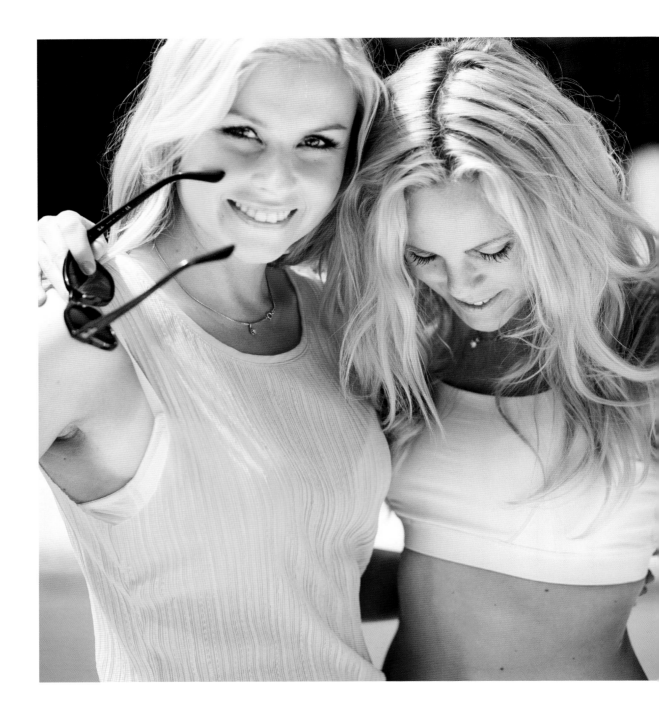

CONTENTS

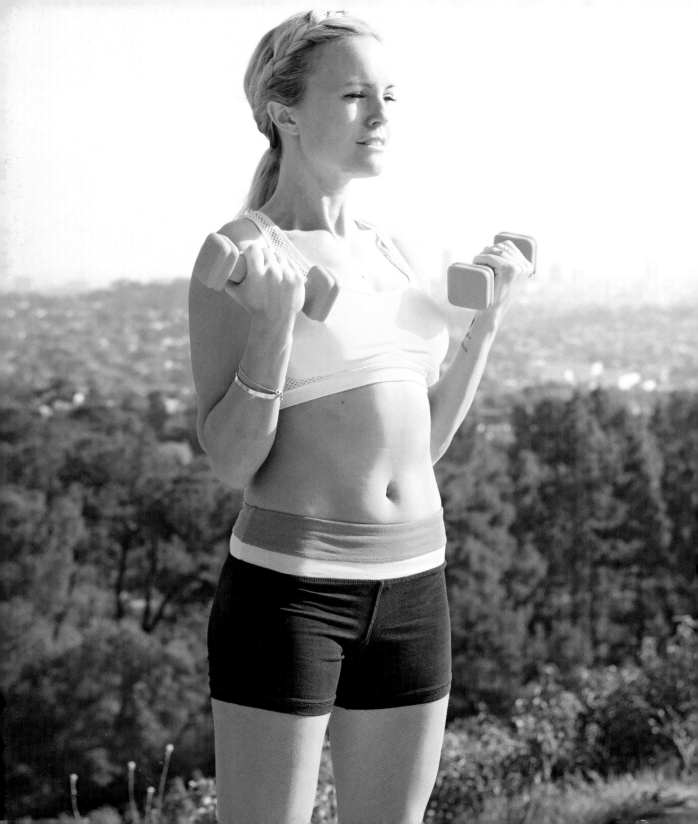

PART 1
FITNESS

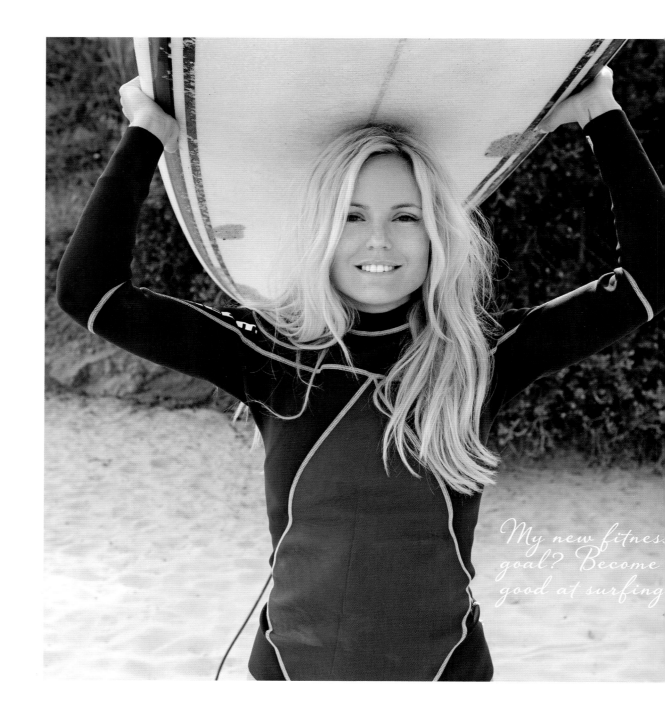

My new fitness goal? Become good at surfing

Sofi Says

Why a fitness book? I've often been asked this question since I started this project. There are, of course, people who know more than I when it comes to exercise (and fashion, for that matter), but I would like to give you my views, my insights, and my inspiration.

I'd like to present healthy ideals and show you how to think right about food and exercise without diets and finger-pointing. You can't just eat however much you want of whatever you want (except cucumbers, maybe), but I don't want to be the kind of person who lives to count calories. Snore. You've got to think smart instead, by following the "don't eat more than you actually need" rule and others that can help you get into a healthy cycle of food and exercise. Do you, like me, live a hectic life and want tips for smart, healthy snacks; exercises for your booty that really work; upbeat exercise music; and motivation collected all into one place? Then this book is for you.

I've never been one for trying all the latest trendy diets, and I think that's what's kept me from messing up my metabolism. Sure, good genes help, but I've always had a healthy attitude toward food and included exercise in my everyday routine. And by exercise, I mean routines that get me to sweat and give me results— I'm no Pilates girl. Just like I love traveling to new places, I also love testing out new workouts, and I love the feeling of sweat drops running down my temples.

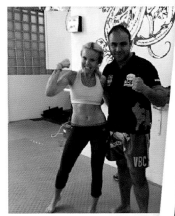

MMA in a Sweaty Gym

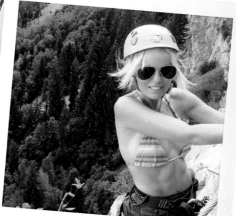

Climbing Outdoors in Chamonix

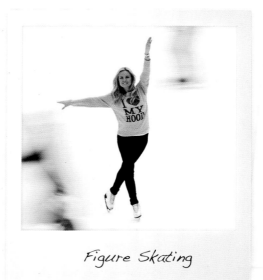

Figure Skating

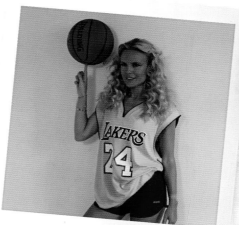

Point Guard

I started my active life at Dalénhallen in Lidingö with a pair of uncomfortable ice skates on my feet. Seven years later, I landed my first double Salchow and shortly thereafter switched to basketball and boys instead. I was a point guard and loved to shoot three-pointers and set up games. I still have my basketball, which now sits in my apartment in New York; when I get a break from my work, I like to head down to the nearest court and dribble for a while. Another thing that's always been close to my heart is skiing. During my last year of high school, I studied to become a ski instructor so that I could work for a season in the Alps after taking my final exams. And now I'm also engaged to a man who lives in the world's best ski resort, Verbier, so loose snow and steep hills are never too far away. Throughout the last ten years I've

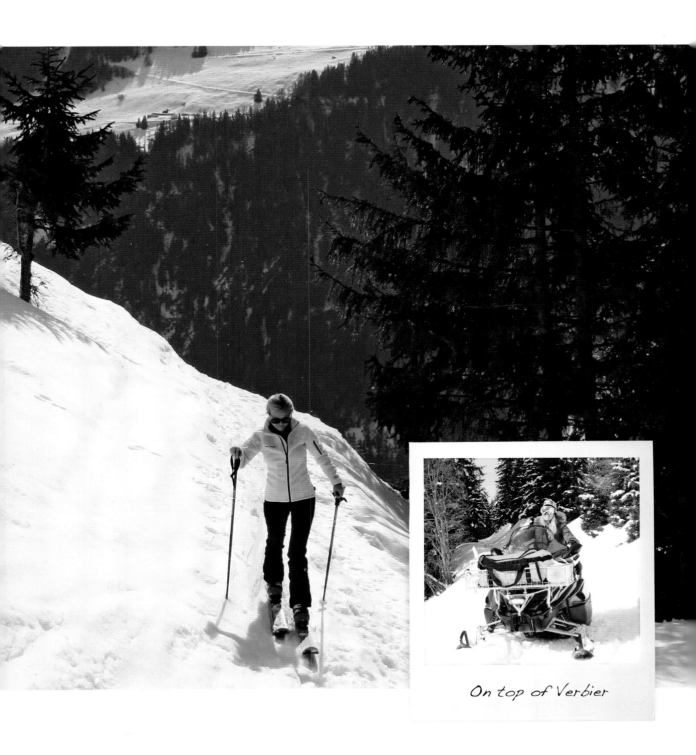

On top of Verbier

tried everything from mountain climbing to pole dancing to waterskiing and running. Variation is what keeps me satisfied.

Kate Moss coined the expression "nothing tastes as good as skinny feels." I think it would be best to replace "skinny" with "strong." After all, if there's anything that's a must for me, it's feeling strong. In my work I'm exposed to stress and pressures every day, and I don't think I could manage my hectic lifestyle if my body wasn't strong. I need energy in order to be able to give energy in my writing and in front of the camera.

I wrote this book together with my colleague, Julia Fors, who is a health and beauty writer. We have, throughout the years, met the world's best trainers—from the guy who whips Victoria's Secret girls into shape so well that they look photoshopped to the girl who's the secret behind Madonna's well-developed biceps. In this book, we've collected all the insider tips we've come across and mixed them with our own personal mottos and secrets.

I would like to be able to look back on my life and be proud of the things that I've done rather than be disappointed about the things that I didn't get to do. That applies to exercise just as much as it does to my outlook on life as a whole. It's never too late to begin a new way of thinking and living.

Enjoy!

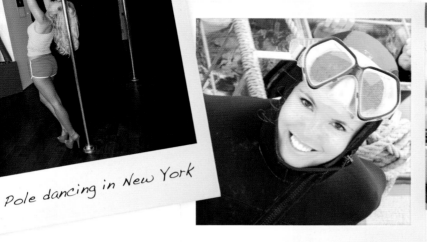

Pole dancing in New York

Diving with sharks outside Cape Town

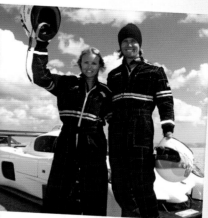

Pedal to the metal at Gotland Ring

"NOTHING TASTES AS GOOD AS STRONG FEELS"

SOFI FAHRMAN

Sofi's Five Most Common Questions from Readers

1. How many times a week do you run, and for how long?
My goal is three times a week; the distance varies from four to eight kilometers, depending on the day. I don't like to put pressure on myself by deciding how far I'm going to run in advance. Doing that makes it all too easy to end up disappointed if I don't have the energy for it. Instead, I use an app on my iPhone to keep track of my pace. I increase my pace on the way home and never push myself too hard in the beginning. Something else I always do is really give 110 percent those last hundred meters so I can have a positive experience and finish when I reach the end—knowing that I had that extra 10 percent to give.

2. You seem to live a stressful life. What do you think when you don't feel like working out?
A little bit is better than nothing at all. The feeling you get when you've gone to the gym or gone running around a track, despite not wanting to, is twice as good as usual when you get back home. Sometimes I'll do a super-short fifteen-minute workout. I've even gone to the gym and done nothing but use the sauna. When things get stressful, I need routines, and just leaving the computer is a reward in and of itself.

3. What do you eat after a workout?
If I'm in a good exercise routine, I've found that protein shakes give the best results. I feel full and get my energy back. I usually blend together milk, a banana, and Herbalife's vanilla-flavored protein shake. Since I usually exercise in the morning, the protein shake is enough for me until lunch.

4. Party princess and working out—how do those go together?
Hahaha. I train the way I party: in moderation. I work out and dance to feel good, and I try to find routines that work well with my body. I ought to add that before I turned thirty, my body was quite forgiving. Now I can't cheat as much. I need sleep, get hungover like everyone else, and am useless at work the day after.

5. Your favorite workout?

Besides sex? I'd have to say anything my body isn't used to. I love to shock it with new things. I'm a curious person, and that crosses over into my outlook on training, too. As soon as I read about a new kind of workout, I'm on it. At the moment, it's SoulCycle and Physique 57 in New York.

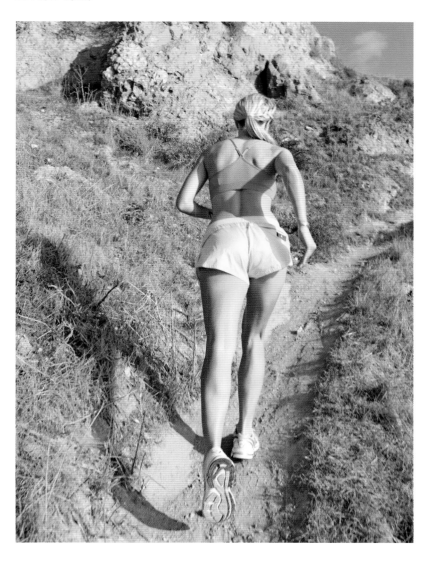

Train insane or remain the same

"The difference between a goal and a dream is a deadline"

Train Smarter

Find your own inspiration to work out

Has it been weeks, months, or even years since you last put your feet in a pair of running shoes? Or is it time to take your normal workout routine to a whole new level and get yourself the dream body you've always wanted? Regardless of where you start, one of the first steps that leads to good results is finding your own personal motivation.

In order for your goal—a toned, strong, beach-ready bikini body—to be realistic, you should already be creating a mental picture of how you want to look and feel when you've achieved your result.

Actors and models have tons of built-in deadlines. These can be revealing romance scenes, red-carpet events, or fashion shows. Many of those we've interviewed throughout the years for *Sofi's mode* have said the same thing—that these deadlines increase their motivation to get results.

What sort of reasons do you have to get into the best shape of your life? Be specific! How do you want to look? How do you want to feel? Which clothes do you want to feel perfectly self-confident wearing? When's your personal deadline? The more specific you are when you make goals for yourself, the easier it'll be to really motivate yourself on those days when you aren't feeling quite so up to it.

Give it twenty-one days

We've made it easy for you and formulated a workout and nutrition program (Bikini Boot Camp, p. 144) that gives you all the tools you need to mold your body and build nice, toned muscles. A strong and healthy body is a sexy body. Strong is the new skinny!

Now it's up to you to put your energy into your workouts. If it's any consolation, even celebrities and models can't pay anybody else to work out for them. Everybody has to put time, sweat, and energy into their workouts. Whatever you do, we'd like you to promise us one thing: that you at least give this program three weeks before getting tired and deciding to begin your new life next week instead. According to research, it takes your body twenty-one days to create or break a habit. After that period of time, it becomes easier to do what you should be doing. On the twenty-second day, the habit is established,

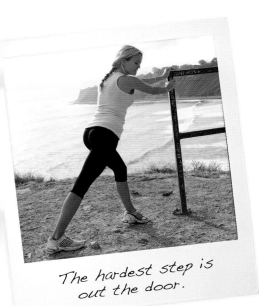

The hardest step is out the door.

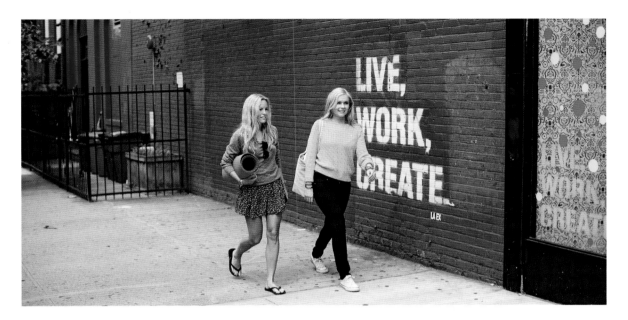

and you'll notice that exercising doesn't feel like such a chore anymore. It'll be as obvious as brushing your teeth.

Another positive side effect of starting to exercise is that you'll actually get addicted to your workout. Yes, it's really true! When you exercise, your body releases dopamine and serotonin, your own feel-good hormones. The more you exercise, the easier it'll be to keep going, since your body will want more of those same good feelings that exercise brings.

Apart from good feelings and a body that is completely strong and sexy, your workouts will also boost your self-confidence. When you exercise, you develop a better body image and automatically feel more satisfied with yourself and your body. And really, what's sexier than exuberant self-confidence?

Work out smarter—not harder

Does a life that includes exercise mean that you have to go to the gym and work out every day? No. Seriously, who has the time for that?

There's nothing that says this is a must to get yourself a healthy, toned body. On top of that, if you lead a hectic life, it's impossible to squeeze in time at the gym each and every day. Our philosophy, and

"The more you exercise, the easier it'll be to keep going"

one that is supported by a number of studies as well as by the best trainers we've met throughout the years, is instead all about training smarter.

As you'll notice, you can do every exercise in this book without once going to the gym. If you train at the gym for more than an hour, you risk not only becoming tired and fatigued but also putting a lot of stress on your body, which causes it to release cortisol. Cortisol builds up when we're stressed, when we train too hard, and when we don't get enough calories in ourselves, and you might say that it's a bodylicious body's worst enemy, as it, among other things, breaks down muscle mass, increases blood sugar levels, and decreases the burning of fat. If you exercise too often and too intensely, your endocrine system won't get a chance to recover, and that's when these kinds of things happen.

By following our training program, which has a perfect balance between high- and low-intensity exercise, along with important rest days, you'll be in the best condition to sculpt the body you want to have without needlessly sacrificing a lot of time.

Add in strength

The most common workout mistakes are focusing only on cardio or constantly going through the same routine without challenging your body to develop. If you constantly go for the same run or go to the

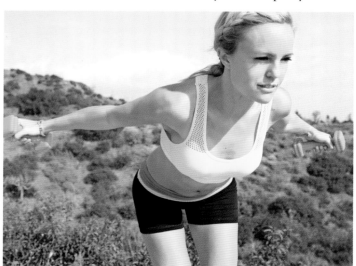

same BodyPump class and wonder why nothing's happening, this is your answer. If you want to decrease your body fat percentage or sculpt your body, you'll have a hard time getting anywhere with cardio alone.

Cardio burns calories when you exercise, but it doesn't do anything to change your metabolism and the total amount of calories that you burn.

If you want to boost your calorie burning, which will keep you naturally slim and toned, the trick is to combine cardio and strength training exercises. After strength training, your body continues to burn energy for up to forty-eight hours. Yes, even when you're sleeping or watching your favorite TV show. The more muscle mass you have, the more fat you'll burn, since muscles use energy even when at rest. Muscles burn three times as much energy as fat does; on top of that, one kilogram of muscles takes up about 20 percent less space in your body than a kilogram of fat, so as a bonus, you'll also look tighter and more toned.

There's a myth that we women will become big and muscular as soon as we begin strength training. This doesn't check out. Women have ten to thirty times lower levels of the hormones responsible for muscle growth than men, which is what stops us from getting "big." On the contrary, our muscles will get harder, sturdier, and more well-defined from strength training.

You're just a workout away from a good mood!

Add in interval training

If you're like us, you're probably always looking for ways to cut down on the time you spend exercising, right? We've got good news! It's entirely possible to get the same effects of one workout in half the time if you train the right way.

Innumerable studies in this field claim that you can get results that are just as good in a shorter amount of time by training more effectively. High-intensity interval training is absolutely the most effective way to burn calories and fat while toning your body quickly.

Interval training is based on the concept of pushing yourself almost to your maximum pulse for short periods of time, then recovering for a little while before bringing up your heart rate once again. You might think of it like sprinting for your heart, which is forced to work harder and thus pump more oxygen into your blood, as well as boosting both your endurance and calorie burning.

Your body is smart, so it always tries to get by with as little energy as possible. If you always work out at a relatively comfortable pace, your body will get used to this after a while and burn fewer calories with the same exercise routine. On the other hand, when you stomp on the gas pedal and sprint in intervals, you force your body's muscles to work harder once more, and thus burn more calories.

PEOPLE WHO ARE PHYSICALLY ACTIVE FEEL MORE IMPASSIONED AND ENTHUSIASTIC COMPARED TO THOSE WHO DON'T EXERCISE.

BODYLICIOUS *tips!*

Use weights that challenge you; the last few repetitions should be heavy, though not impossible to complete. Always rest one to two days between high-intensity interval training workouts. If you do the bikini program (p. 74–81), for example, do it on Mondays, Wednesdays, and Fridays.

Interval training is especially good for running, where you can alternate between jogging and a fast run. You can also perform a series of high-intensity exercises in quick succession, like in our Bikini Boot Camp (p. 149). To challenge you even more, we've put together this workout called Tabata interval training, often described as the world's most effective training. The workout is short but unbelievably effective.

Add in combined sets

To push your body further still to its maximum capacity, we've also designed our training program with combined sets, which bring quicker results. By combining two exercises into one, you not only halve your workout time but the exercises also become more effective compared to doing each one individually.

In other words: you'll burn more calories and get a stronger, more sculpted body in a shorter period of time. What's more, you won't get bored!

A Bodylicious fat-burning secret

If your personal goal is to lose weight, we have a Bodylicious trick just for you. And best of all, we promise that it'll give you the guaranteed result!

To burn fat most effectively, you should either do interval training workouts and keep your heart rate as close to your maximum as possible, or opt for low-intensity (about 50 to 60 percent of your maximum pulse) training. Then your body won't take so much energy from the glycogen in your muscles, but rather from fat deposits. A perfect example of low-intensity training is going for a walk. The best fat-burning exercise is a walk in the morning, before you've eaten breakfast—that'll give you 10 to 20 percent better fat burning.

Why? Your body prefers to use carbohydrates as energy sources; that is, the energy from the food you just ate. When you take a walk on an empty stomach, your body is forced to instead use your fat reserves directly as energy.

Getting up, drinking a glass of water (or perhaps a cup of coffee), and then going out and walking for thirty to forty-five minutes is very effective. It might feel like a chore to walk without having eaten breakfast, but it's actually a matter of habit. When you start getting into it, you might even begin to feel that you enjoy starting the day with a walk with good music in your ears. Morning walks are also a great way to find time to structure your thoughts before the day is underway, and on top of that, breakfast will taste especially good afterward!

Avoid training

Never train when you have a fever, a sore throat, or joint pain, or if you feel extremely tired. It can be harmful to work out even with a mild infection in your body. It's also a complete waste of time, since all your energy is going to your immune system in order to fight off the virus. If, however, you've just got a bit of a cold or are feeling somewhat off, you can try some light exercise. If you're not sure, rest a day or two and then start up again.

What about post-workout aches?

Did your monster glute workout live up to its name the day after? Sorry—that's no excuse to skip your workout. In fact, some light exercise can actually help to ease some of the pain. Be careful not to overwork tired muscles, and focus on muscle groups other than the sore ones. Swimming, yoga, Pilates, and light walks are good ways to exercise when you're sore after a workout.

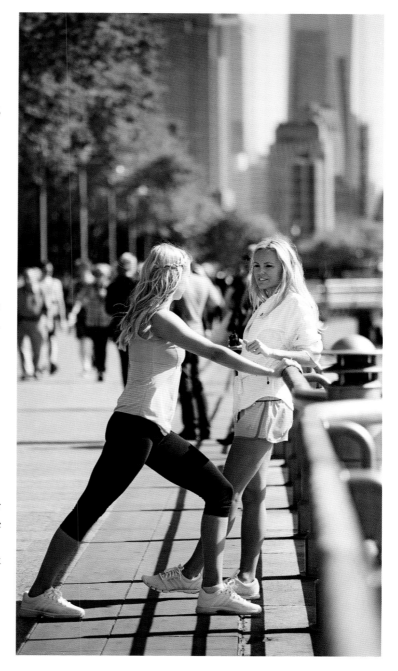

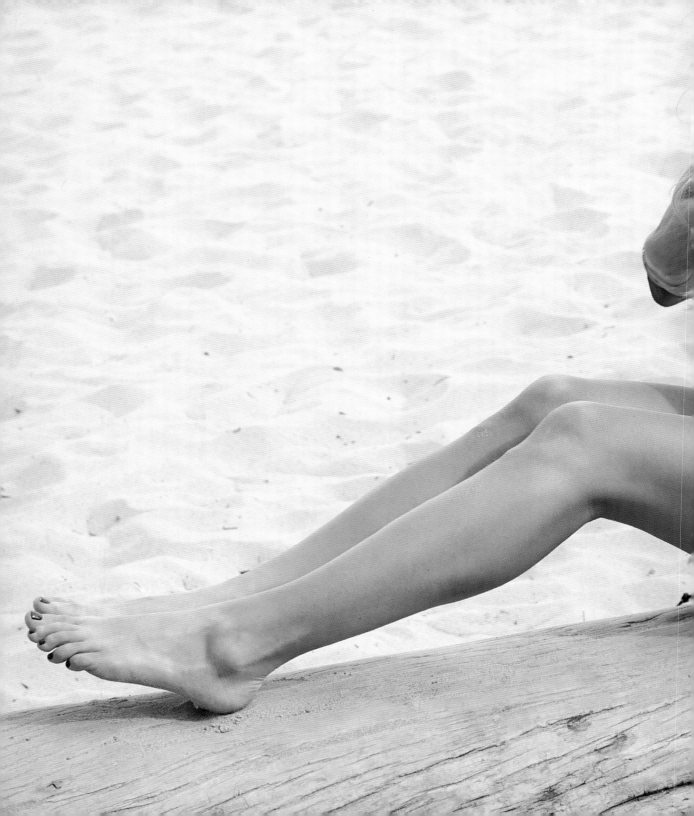

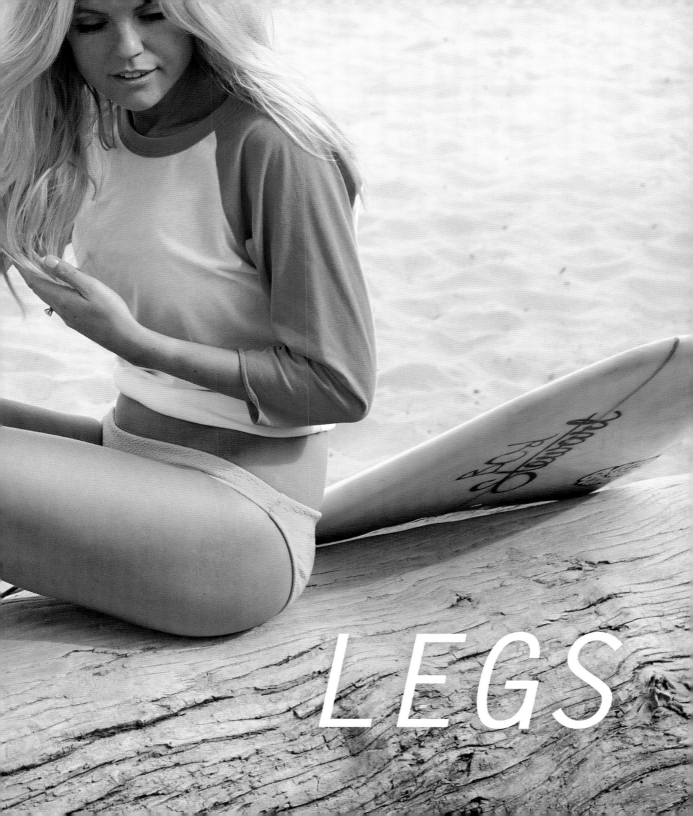

LEGS

LEGS »

As soon as I put up a picture on the blog showing me out and about in a dress or a pair of jean shorts, the questions come in: how do I train my legs? Here comes my answer.

There are no shortcuts. No, don't put the book down now. My recipe for good-looking legs is a mix of running and plain leg exercises. Throughout the years I've taken friends, colleagues, and boyfriends out for runs. I've even been on a date with a pair of running shoes on. I love the combination of working out and socializing, so I usually set the pace such that I can run and carry on a conversation at the same time. Sitting down for a coffee break for a few hours and gossiping over a latte isn't my thing; I'd rather head out to West Side Highway or Central Park and go through the weekend's adventure.

I often hear people say "I don't have time to exercise!" This is an excuse I don't buy. At times I've juggled three jobs at once: writing books, writing for the paper, and hosting a TV show. But I swear I have always had time for a short run—twenty minutes is better than nothing. I don't need to set aside any great amount of time; I simply lace up my shoes as soon as I get a break. For me, it's usually a morning thing; the longer the day runs, the harder I find it to get that sort of opening. And I don't want to be the kind of person who cancels a nice dinner date in order to go out running.

At the same time, running is the solution when I'm out traveling around a lot. I don't need a gym or any equipment. I don't even know how many places I've seen and discovered just going out for a run. A sunrise at one of the world's most beautiful beaches in Tulum, a residential area in Austin, picturesque views in Camps Bay, and even London's heated morning traffic. I've seen a good deal with my running shoes on.

And now, to my exercises. These are great for runners and walkers alike. Here we go!

BODYLICIOUS *tip!*

To give your calf and thigh muscles an extra work out, run up and down for the hills. Even the slightest hill makes the workout more intense. The mountainous hiking area Runyon Canyon in Los Angeles is a favorite place for power-walking celebrities like Cameron Diaz, Lauren Conrad, and Jessica Biel.

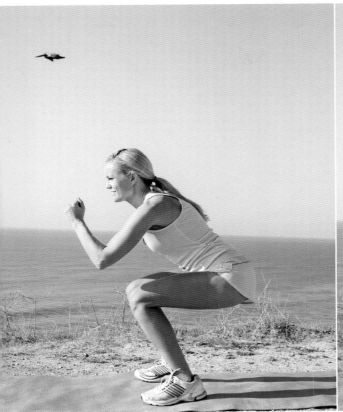
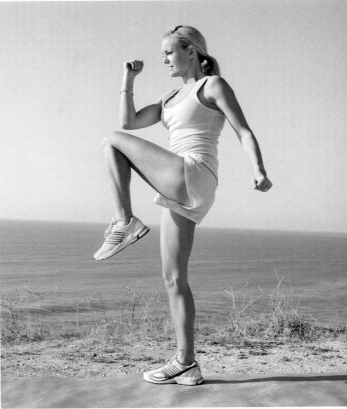

SQUAT WITH LIFT

Stand with your legs hip width apart. Come down into a deep squat, and as you come up, lift your left knee up to your right elbow. Come down into a squat once more, and now lift your right knee up to your left elbow. Perform thirty squats with lifts.

"This exercise is a good warm-up since it'll get you breathing a bit more heavily. We do it a lot, especially before a Victoria's Secret show, since it tones the muscles in your legs very well. You can also fasten small weights around your ankles to get some extra strength training for your legs," said Hollywood personal trainer Justin Gelband, when I met and trained with him in New York.

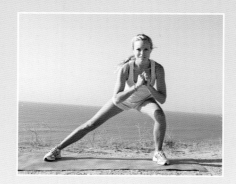

2

SIDE LUNGE
WITH HOP

Stand with your legs hip width apart with your
hands together in front of your chest. Take a long
step to the side with your left leg and bend your
left knee, coming down into a deep lunge. Keep
your right leg straight. Press your left leg back
to the starting position, balance on your right
leg, and take three small hops on your right leg.
Come out to the side again and perform twelve
repetitions, then repeat on the other side for a
total of twenty-four repetitions.

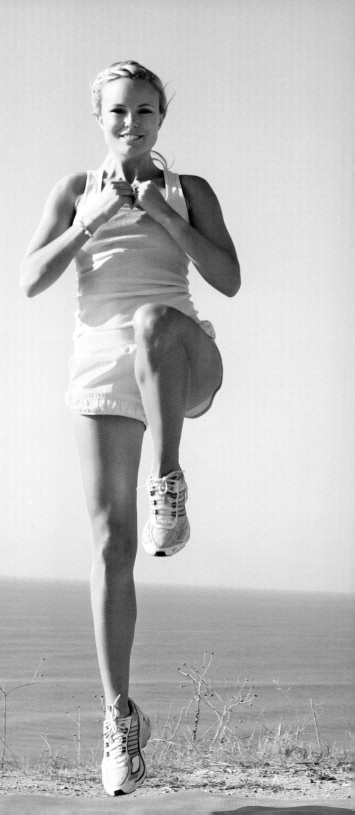

SINGLE LEG SQUAT

Stand with your legs hip width apart. Lift your right leg a few inches from the ground and bring down your body as if you were going to sit on a chair. Here, it's important that you really push your booty backward and out and make sure that the knee of your standing leg doesn't come so far forward as to obscure your toes. Tighten your stomach and keep your leg stretched, but right as you reach the imaginary "chair," come back up in a controlled manner. Perform six squats on each leg for a total of twelve squats.

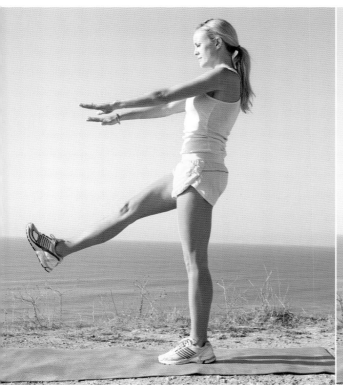

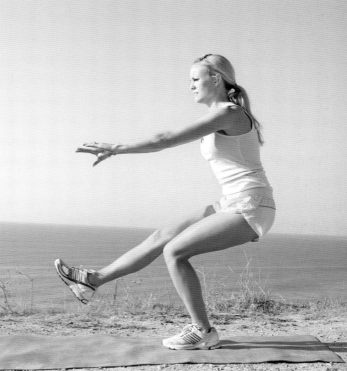

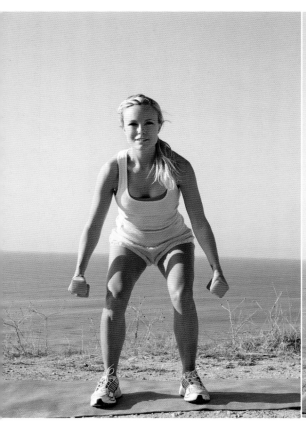
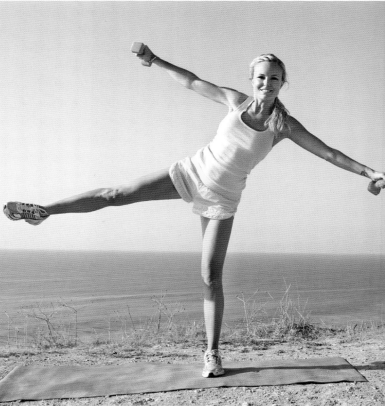

SQUAT WITH STAR

A whole-body exercise that works your shoulders, arms, thighs, core, and booty. The exercise is especially toning for the area where your bikini meets your booty, and tightens up anything loose.

Stand with your legs shoulder width apart, a dumbbell in each hand. Come down into a deep squat, as if you were about to sit on a chair. When you come up, lift the right leg straight out to the side while lifting your arms out to the sides so that the weights come up to shoulder height. Come down into a squat again and repeat on the other leg. Perform twelve stars on each side for a total of twenty-four stars.

CURTSY LUNGE

Stand with your legs hip width apart, hands on your hips. Bring up your chest and relax your shoulders. Bring your right leg behind your left leg and bend both knees so your right leg is nearly parallel to the ground. Return to the starting position and repeat with the other leg. Repeat twelve times on each leg for a total of twenty-four lunges.

Tip!
Lunges are absolutely the most effective exercise to tone your booty and thighs.

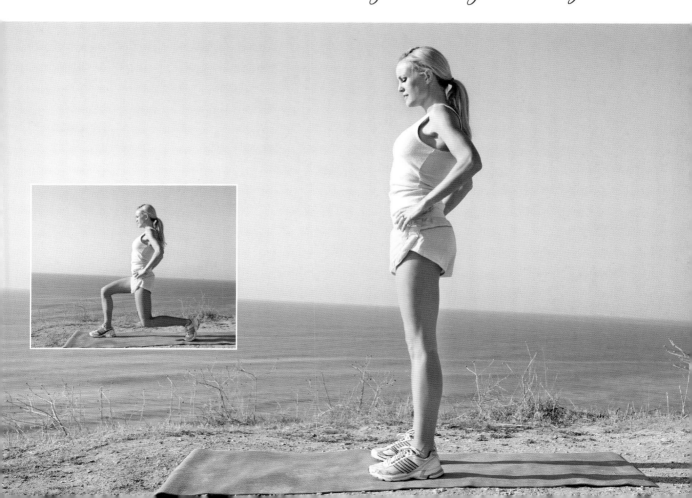

UPWARD-FACING BOOTY PRESS

Lie down on a mat with your knees bent, palms down. Tighten your core, booty, and thighs and press up your booty so you have a straight line from your knees to your shoulders. While doing this, lift one leg and flex the foot, pressing it up as if you're trying to reach the roof. Perform twelve flexed-foot lifts, returning the foot to the mat each time, before repeating with the other leg for a total of twenty-four lifts.

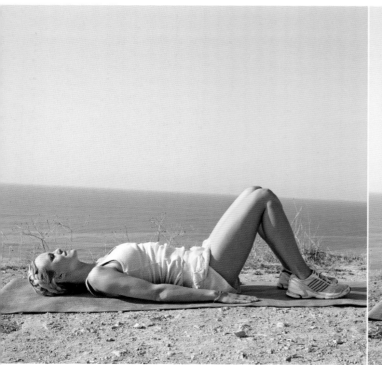
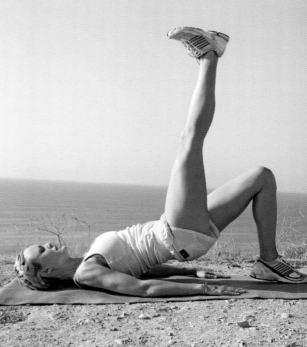

LEG OVERVIEW»

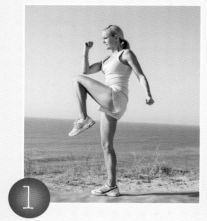

SQUAT WITH LIFT
X 30

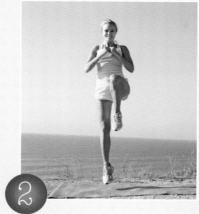

SIDE LUNGE WITH HOP
X 24

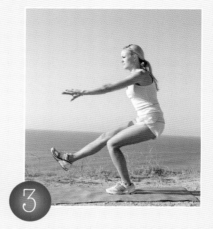

SINGLE LEG SQUAT
X 12

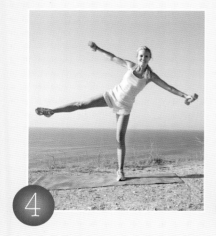

SQUAT WITH STAR *X 24*

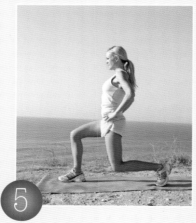

CURTSY LUNGE *X 24*

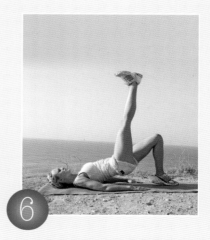

UPWARD-FACING BOOTY PRESS *X 24*

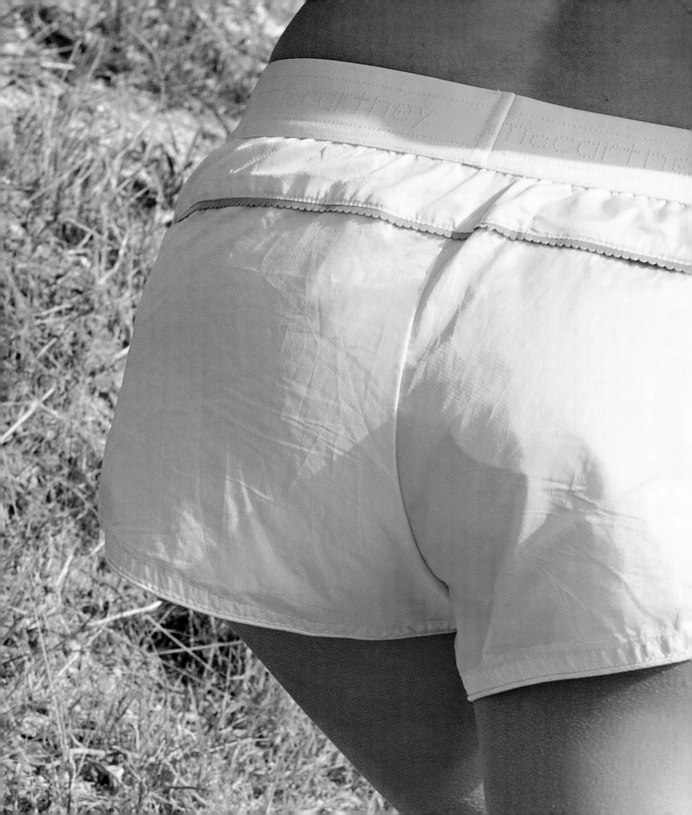

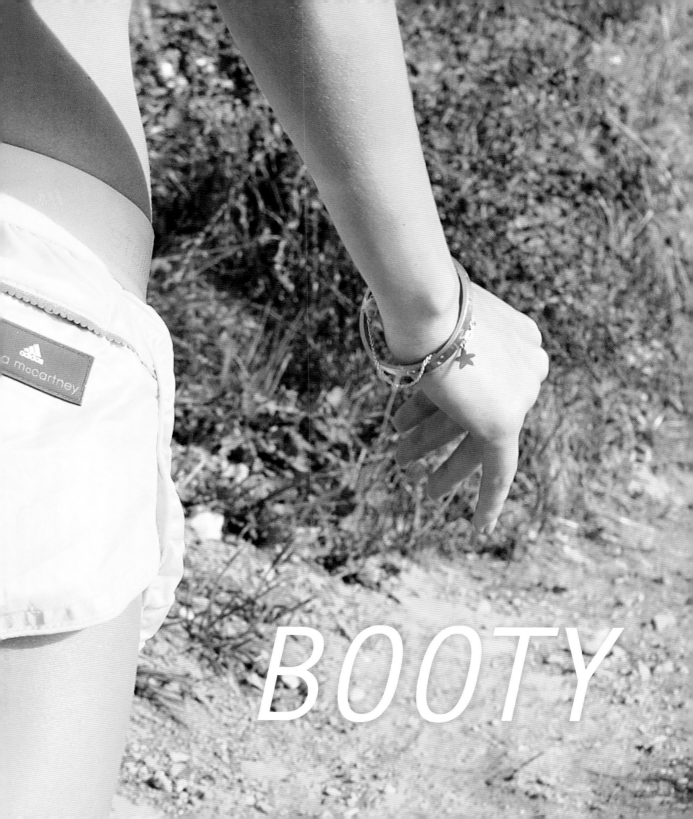

BOOTY

BOOTY »

Of all the celebrity trainers I've interviewed and sweated alongside throughout the years, I have an obvious favorite—David Kirsch. Why?

Hold on tight—he's known as "the assmaster." You really can't help but trust a guy like that. Right?

Karolina Kurkova, a model, was the one who began calling him "the master of the ass" after he remodeled her booty with the help of the right exercises. After that, he trademarked the name in the United States. In an interview he said, for example, that he sees himself as a sculptor when it comes to the booty. He says that there isn't a single booty in the world that he can't lift, tone, build up, slim down, make rounder, tighten up, or make cheekier.

I remember thinking that this sounded too good to be true. But after having tested his exercises, I was more than happy to be a part of them. When I combine running with his exercises, I really notice the results. Your booty really does get a lift.

We women are preprogrammed to store fat around our booties, hips, and thighs. Sure, it's unfair, but that doesn't mean there's no toning up these areas. As I'm sure you already know, spot reduction does not work and never will. But you absolutely can spotsculpt, as Kirsch calls it.

Since the largest muscle group is in your booty, making it a proper calorie burner, the new muscles will also increase your body's overall burning of fat and calories. I've learned that variety is really key here. A single exercise for your booty isn't going to give you the best results; it's not quite that easy. There are three muscles to your booty: the gluteus maximus, medius, and minimus, so to shape and slim, you need to attack it from each and every angle.

My favorite exercise is the "sumo kick," one of the exercises I learned from none other than the "assmaster" himself. You'll find the others here too. Enjoy!

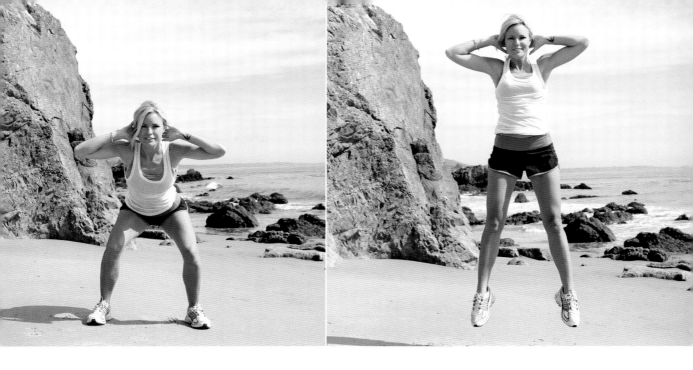

SQUAT WITH JUMP

Stand with your feet just a bit wider than shoulder width apart, feet pointed slightly outward and hands on the back of the neck. Bend your knees while bringing your body down until your thighs are parallel with the ground. Jump straight up into the air. Return to the starting position and repeat twelve times.

Tip!
Work out in the morning and you'll be filled with energy that lasts the whole day.

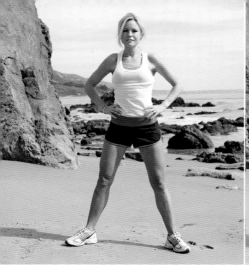 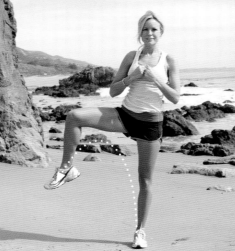 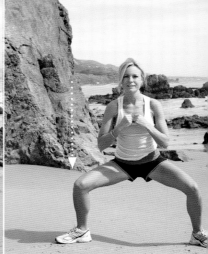

SUMO KICK

This is an easy exercise that doesn't require any sort of special equipment, so you can do it at work, in the living room, or wherever. What's more, it helps to both tone your muscles and slim your thighs.

"The sumo kick is Heidi Klum's favorite exercise," says David Kirsch.

Stand with your feet wide. Lift your right leg from the knee and rotate it to the side in a half-moon. Set the foot down and come down into a medium-depth squat; channel your inner sumo wrestler! When you come up from the squat, lift your right leg again and kick it out with the heel to the side as if you were going to kick an opponent. Repeat this exercise with the left leg. Perform twenty-four sumo kicks, twelve with each leg.

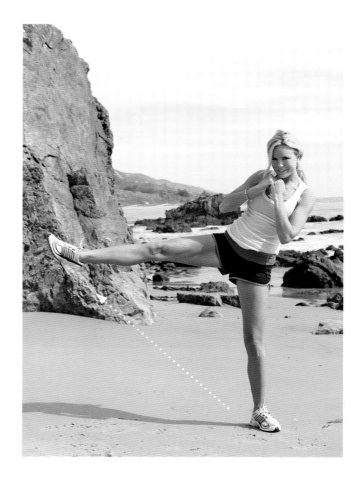

TOE PLIÉ LUNGE

This exercise works your inner thighs and the lower portion of your booty above all. Yep, exactly where we want to feel it! Models often do this exercise before going out on the catwalk, as it instantly gives the booty a tighter look.

Come into a classic squat position with your legs apart, feet turned outward in a 45-degree angle so that your knees and feet are in line with each other. Tighten your booty and come down while you lift your heels from the ground, standing on your toes. Hold the position for two seconds and feel the stretch in your calves; then bring your heels back to the ground while remaining in the same low position. Repeat twelve times.

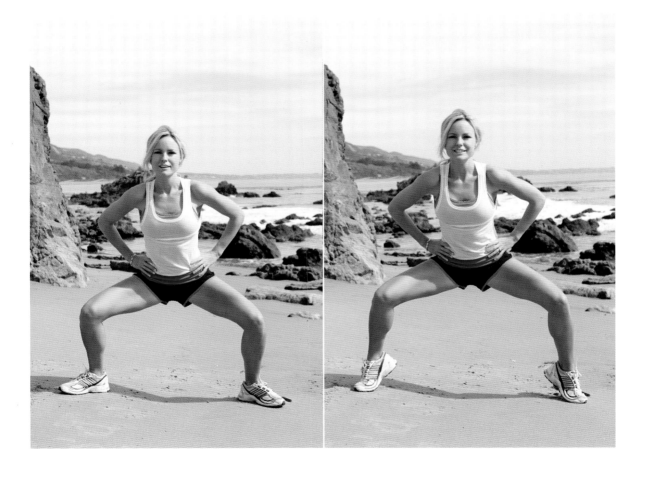

REVERSE LUNGE KICK

Stand with your legs slightly narrower than shoulder width apart, hands clenched into fists in front of your chest. Step back with one leg in a lunge. When you return to the start position, continue bringing the leg forward into a high kick in front of you. Return to the start and repeat with the other leg. Perform twelve kicks with each leg for a total of twenty-four.

"This exercise works all the hip flexor muscles and gives a beautifully sculpted booty and thighs," Marco Borges, Beyoncé's trainer, said when we interviewed him for *Sofi's Mode*.

Develop the right assitude!

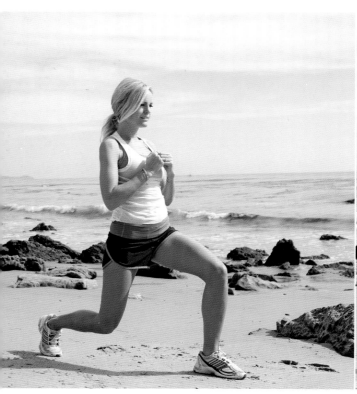

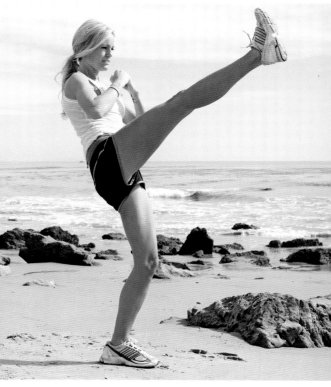

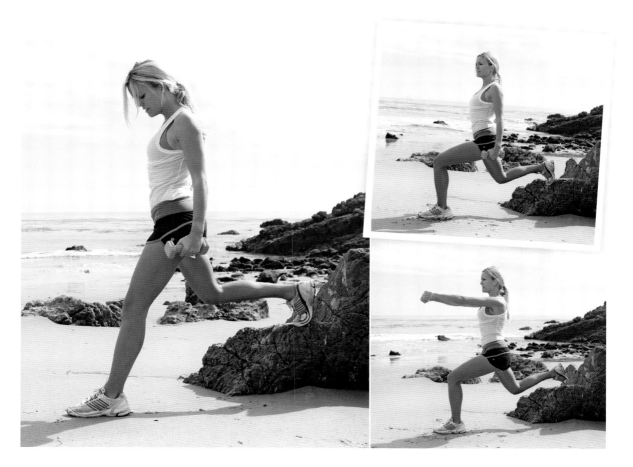

SPLIT SQUAT

Stand with your back to a bench, stool, or other support and hold a water bottle or dumbbell in each hand against your chest. Swing your right leg behind you and place the foot against the chair or other support. Hold in your core and stretch your back as you sink down into a controlled squat without bringing your knee in front of your toes. Bring the weights straight out in front of you with straight arms. Press up to the starting position and repeat twelve times on each leg for a total of twenty-four squats.

BOOTY PRESS

Kneel down on all fours on a mat with your elbows supporting you. Tighten your core and lift your left knee to your chest before pressing it back and lifting it as high as you can. Imagine pushing the ceiling up with your foot. Bring the leg into your chest again and perform twelve repetitions before switching legs for a total of twenty-four repetitions.

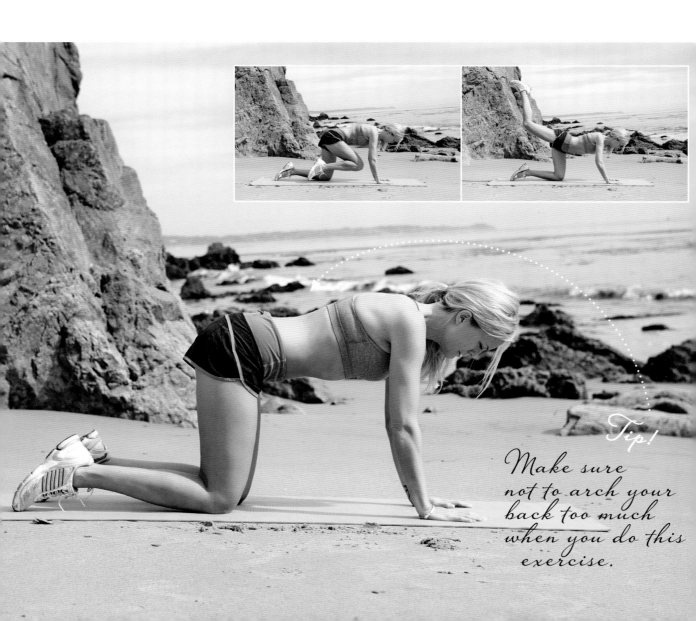

Tip!

Make sure not to arch your back too much when you do this exercise.

BOOTY OVERVIEW»

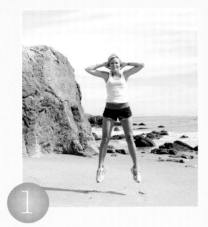

① SQUAT WITH JUMP *X 12*

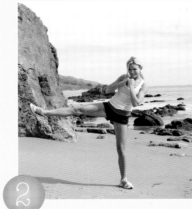

② SUMO KICK *X 24*

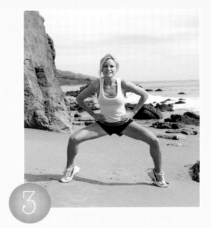

③ TOE PLIÉ LUNGE *X 12*

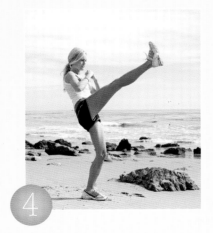

④ REVERSE LUNGE KICK *X 24*

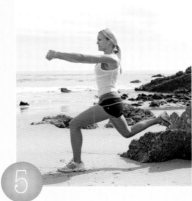

⑤ SPLIT SQUAT *X 24*

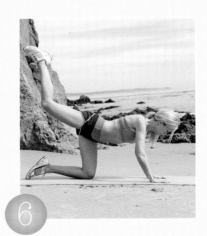

⑥ BOOTY PRESS *X 24*

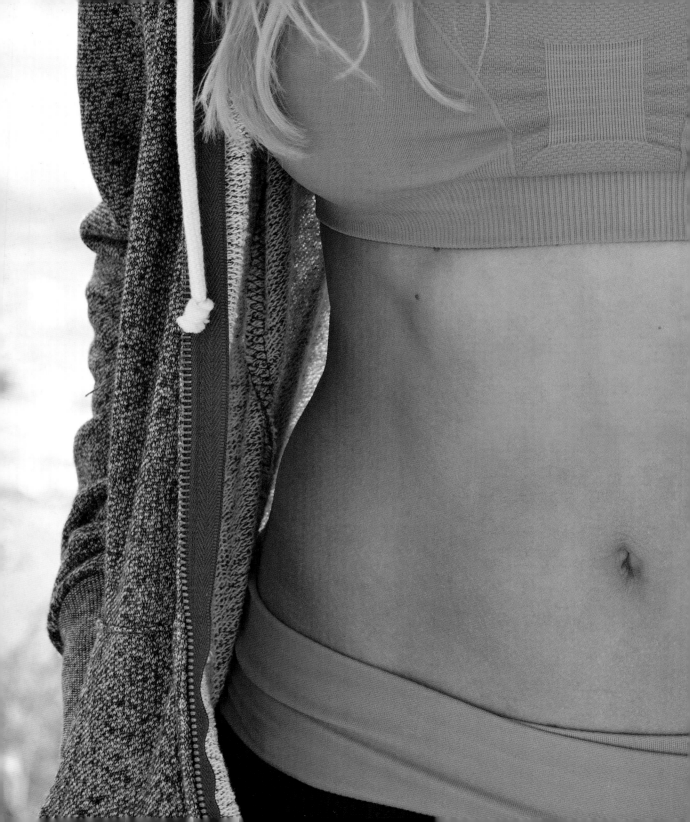

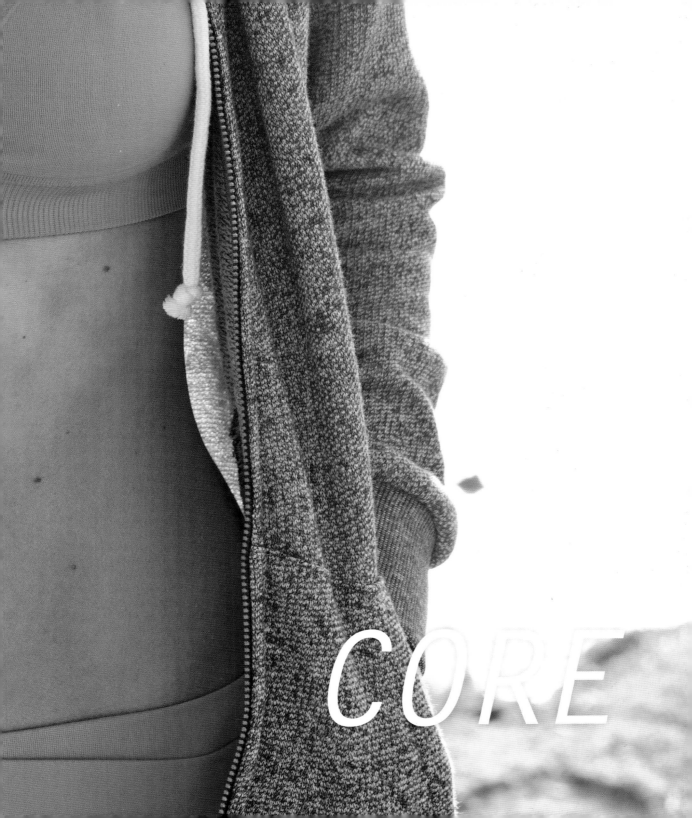

CORE

CORE»

Magical! There's no part of your body that's more fun to have in good shape or one that'll make you look more fit than a toned core. But how do you replace a one-pack with a six-pack? And what do you do when your jeans start to squeeze your waist and make you feel like a muffin? The lazy option is to go to the nearest jeans store and say hello to the next-largest size. Our Bodylicious option is to combine healthy eating with fat-burning workouts using the right exercises.

Why should you train your core? Unlike your arms and legs, your core gets its support from muscles, not from your skeleton. Many find it especially easy to gain weight around the stomach, and for women, this fat is more dangerous than that stored in the thighs and booty, since it releases a substance that increases one's risk for diseases of the heart and circulatory system. And by training your core muscles, you'll improve your posture, which both looks good and gives an impression of fitness.

I myself have always loved core workouts. The more of a chore it feels like, the better. Having a strong core is like having a perfect foundation: it'll help you in all your other workouts. Work your core often and mix up your exercises; try doing them on your back, on your stomach, and on your sides. You'll enjoy it more and will manage more repetitions before your muscles become tired. My favorite exercises are the plank and side plank since I can feel things happening. There's no fuss, and it burns like hell. The best thing about exercises like these is that you don't need a gym. I usually finish a run with a round of these, three periods of one minute each. There's nothing that leaves you feeling more satisfied after your workout than this, I promise! If it's tough and uncomfortable, you're going to get results; it's as simple as that.

Now for my favorite core exercises. When it gets tiring and strenuous, just think of the results!

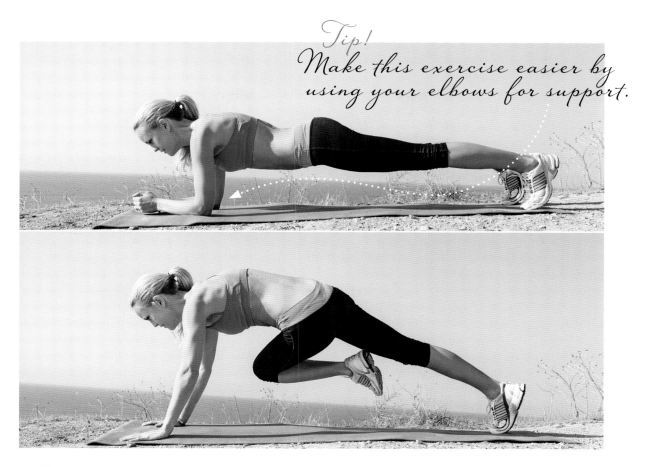

Tip!
Make this exercise easier by using your elbows for support.

MOUNTAIN CLIMBER

Begin in the plank position with straight arms and hands, feet shoulder width apart. Tighten your core, lower your booty, and bring your right knee, rotated outward, in toward your stomach. Bring it back again and continue with the left leg, being careful not to lift your booty too much and lose the strong posture of the core. Perform twenty-five of these leg-to-chest sweeps.

"Many models perform this exercise before photo shoots and fashion shows. It helps the body to look more toned," says trainer Justin Gelband.

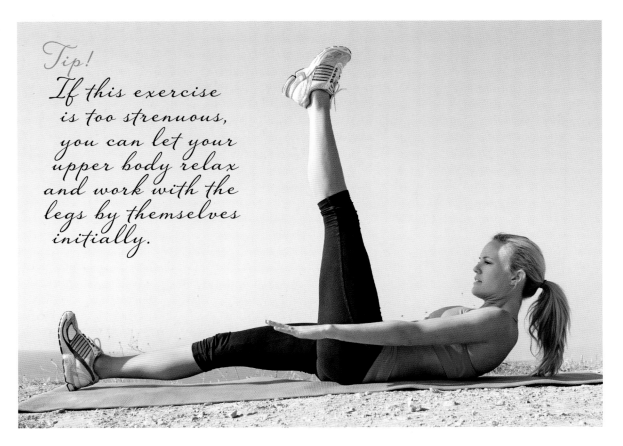

Tip!
If this exercise is too strenuous, you can let your upper body relax and work with the legs by themselves initially.

SCISSORS

Besides working your core muscles—that is, the six pack—you'll also be working your hips, booty, and legs.

Lie on your back with your legs out, arms at your sides. Stretch one leg up into the air at a 90-degree angle so your legs form an L while lifting your head, shoulders, and arms so that your arms are horizontal and about four inches off the ground. Press your lower back into the mat and focus on keeping both legs perfectly straight. Slowly alternate bringing up your left leg and your right leg, like a pair of scissors, keeping the core tight. Count each scissor movement and perform twenty-five repetitions.

3

PLANK

Lie on your stomach and raise your body in a straight line so that the weight of your body rests on your toes and elbows. Hold your hips up and tighten the core muscles, but make sure to continue breathing normally. Maintain this position for one minute. If you feel that your back is beginning to drop, try bringing the time down to thirty seconds and work your way up from there.

Tip!
Bring down your booty and pull your belly button in toward your spine. Remember not to arch your back!

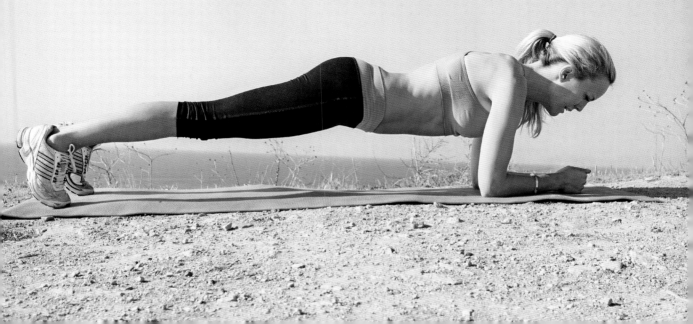

SIDE PLANK

Lie on your side, using your elbow for support. Lift your hips until your body is straight and your elbow is directly beneath your shoulders. Draw in your core and be careful not to tip backward or forward. Lift your free arm, stretching it straight up. Remain in this position for forty seconds before switching sides and repeating the exercise.

Tip!
If this exercise feels too heavy or wobbly, you can keep your free arm along your body instead.

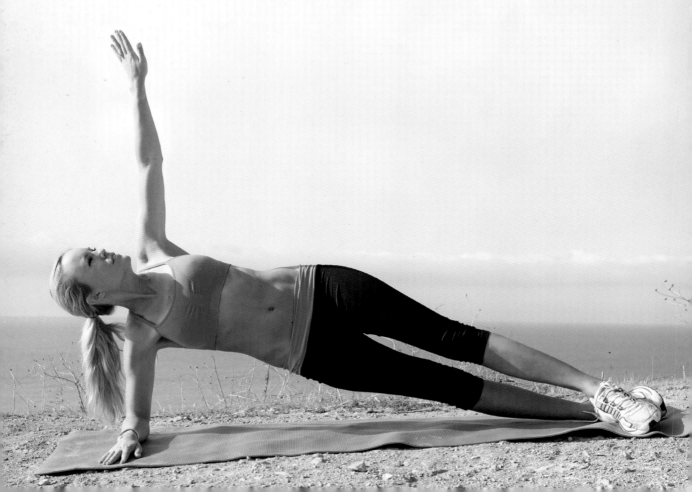

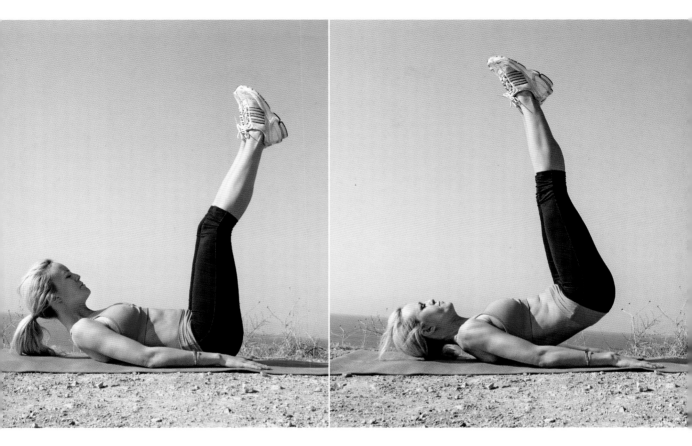

5 HEELS TO THE SKIES

Lie on your back with your legs straight up, forming a 90-degree angle with the ground. Lift your head and upper back. Tighten your core and lift your booty and heels toward the sky, then bring them down slowly. Avoid cheating by pressing down with your arms—lift as much as you can using your core. Perform twenty-five upward pulses.

Tip!

These reverse sit-ups engage your lower core and do away with that stubborn paunch that can otherwise be difficult to get rid of.

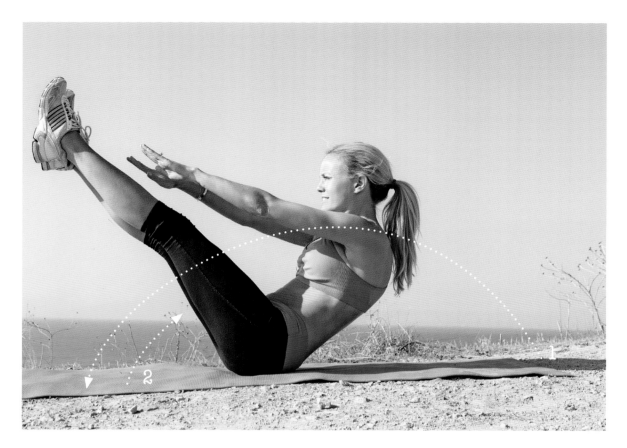

FULL JACKKNIFE SIT-UPS

Lie down on your back, legs straight out and arms at your sides. Tighten your core and come up to touch your toes with your fingers (arrow 1). As you come down, lift your legs up and pulse upward with your upper body, like a folding knife (arrow 2). Come back down to the starting position. This is one repetition; perform twelve.

CORE OVERVIEW»

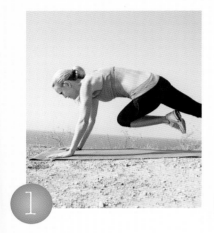

1

MOUNTAIN CLIMBER
X 25

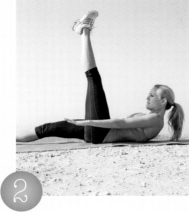

2

SCISSORS *X 25*

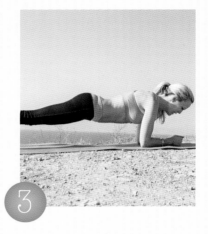

3

PLANK *30 SECONDS*

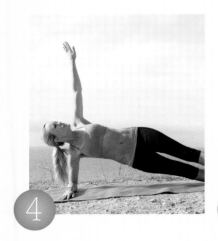

4

SIDE PLANK *40 SECONDS*

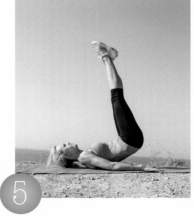

5

**HEELS TO THE
SKIES** *X 25*

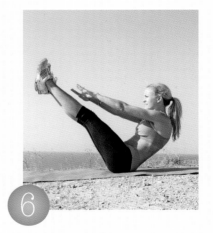

6

**FULL JACKKNIFE
SIT-UPS** *X 12*

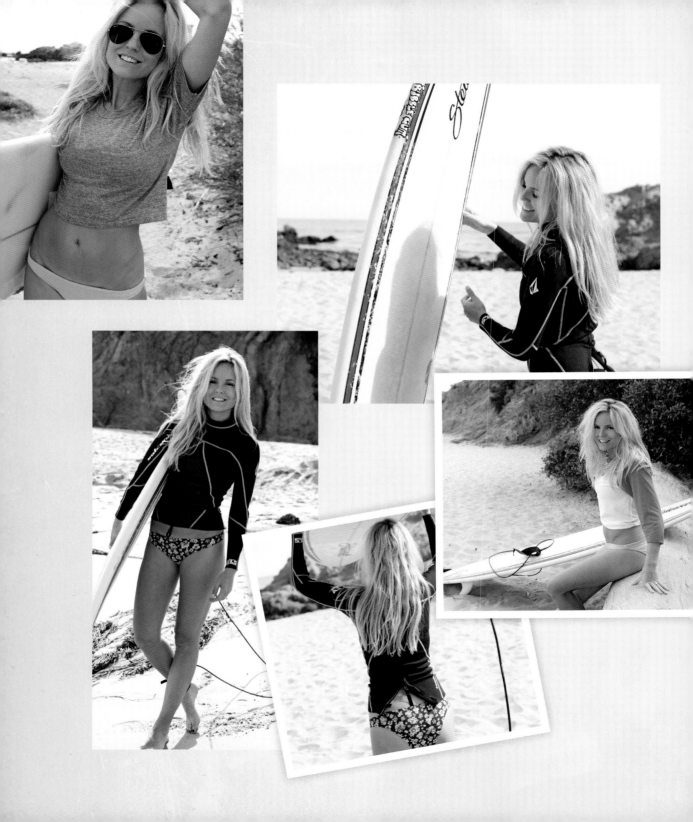

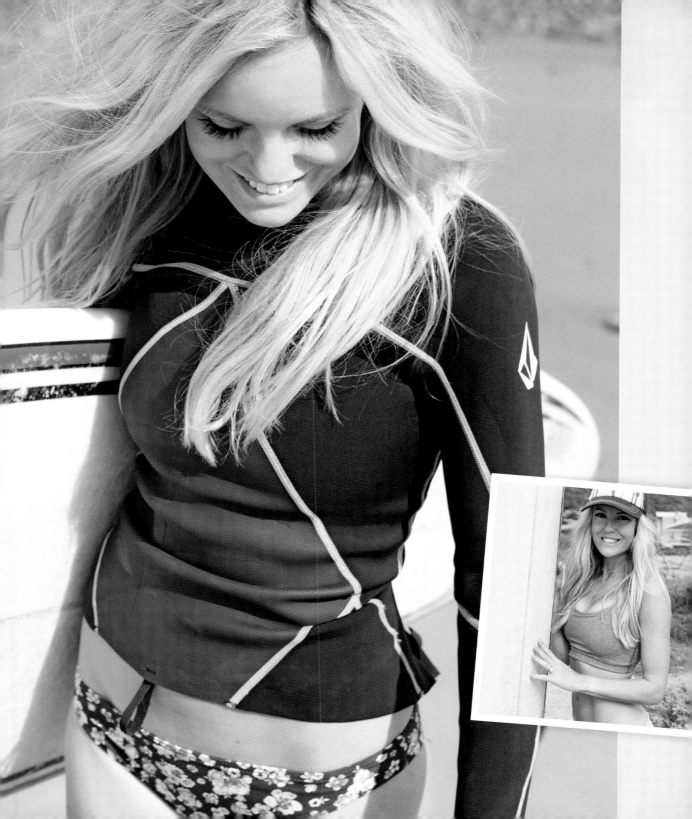

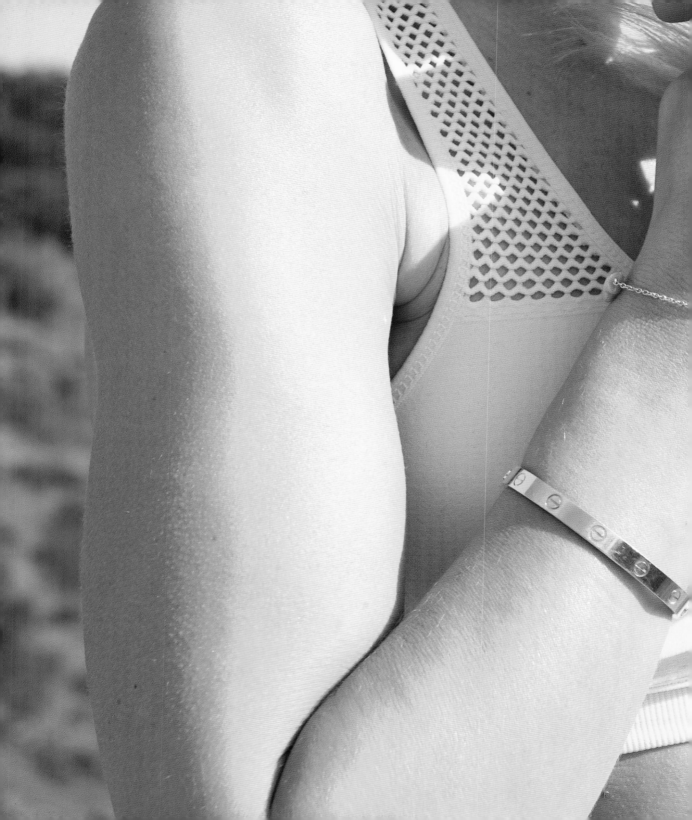

ARMS
AND
SHOULDERS

ARMS AND SHOULDERS »

When we're talking arms and training, there's one star whose name always seems to come up. It seems as if she's just as well known for her well-trained arms as she is for danceable super-hits. I am, of course, talking about Madonna. Impressive, absolutely. Hard work, sure. But attractive? Not so much. Having bigger arms than my fiancé isn't exactly something I'm working toward.

On the other hand, it was incredibly exciting to meet Madonna's trainer, Tracy Anderson, in her studio in New York. After a number of queries, she finally agreed to an interview. With clients like Gwyneth Paltrow, Shakira, and Madonna, she must have something special, no?

And yes, what a bundle of energy! Full of inspiration and a cool outlook on fitness. Lazy scoundrels who complain they aren't getting any results are her worst enemies. She gave me these three tips:

1. Train in the heat

Working out in a warm room makes your body burn more calories and fat. Tracy always makes sure the gym is warmed to at least eighty degrees Fahrenheit.

2. Use light weights

Think lighter weights and more variation. Tracy usually recommends that her clients perform sixty repetitions with weights of around three pounds.

3. Don't forget your triceps

Lots of people focus only on their biceps, but you shouldn't forget your triceps. The triceps muscles make up 60 percent of the total mass of your upper arms, while the biceps only make up 30 percent.

I know it's easy to focus more on your thighs, booty, and core. But well-defined arms make you look fit and healthy. Thin model arms aren't my thing; I want to see the contours.

BODYLICIOUS tip!

When I'm working out at a gym, I always like to end my workout with some time on the rowing machine.

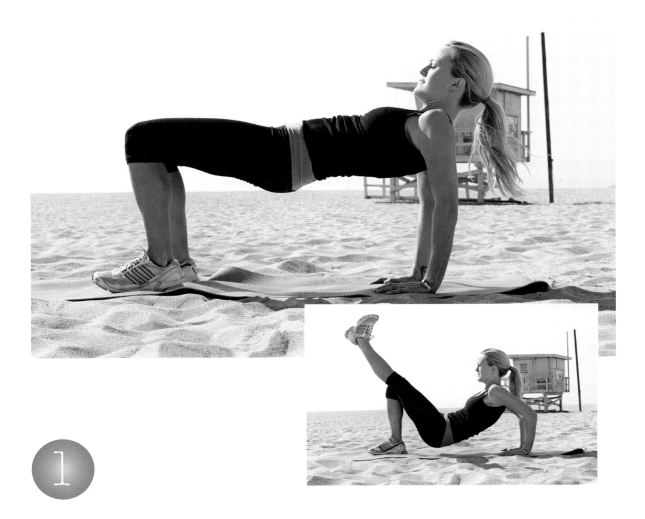

1

TRICEPS DIPS

Sit on the ground with your knees bent upward, your feet a little bit in front of you. Place your hands down with your fingers facing forward. Press yourself up so you stand like a table. Keep a steady position and bend your arms until your elbows reach a 90-degree angle while lifting your right leg and stretching it out in front of you. Press yourself back up to straight arms, releasing the leg back down. Take another dip, but stretch out the left leg before returning to the table position again. Perform six lifts with each leg for a total of twelve dips.

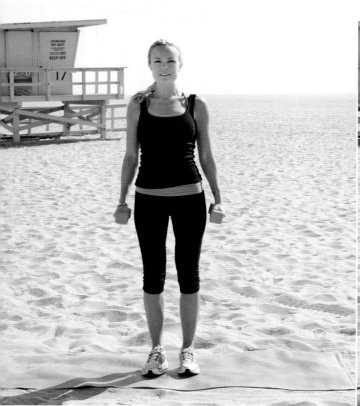
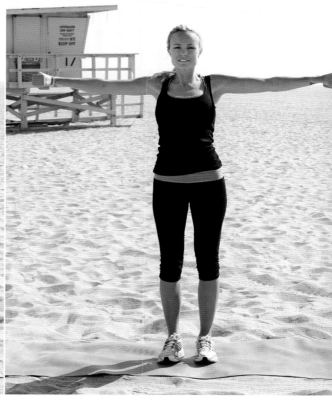

② SHOULDER FLY

Stand with your legs hip width apart, a dumbbell in each hand. Lift both arms straight out to the sides until they reach shoulder height; don't go farther up! Release your arms back down and perform fifteen lifts. Rest a few seconds before doing fifteen more for a total of thirty.

Tip!
Remember to draw your shoulder blades back, and use rather heavy weights.
Those last few reps should be tough!

PLANK WITH DUMBBELL ROWS

This exercise works with your shoulders' stability and all of your core muscles.

Place a couple of dumbbells or water bottles on a mat in front of you. Come into the plank position with your hands right under your shoulders, and place all your weight on your left arm as you lift the weight with your right hand, drawing it up against the right side of your body. Repeat on the other side. Perform six repetitions on each side for a total of twelve.

Tip! *Make sure to keep your shoulder blades together as you lift the weights.*

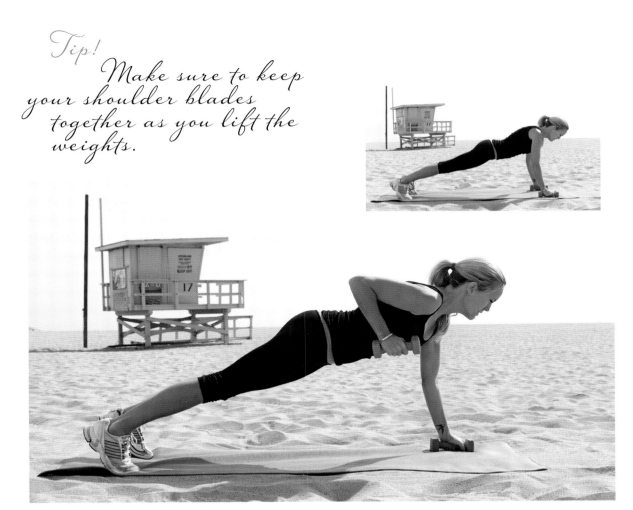

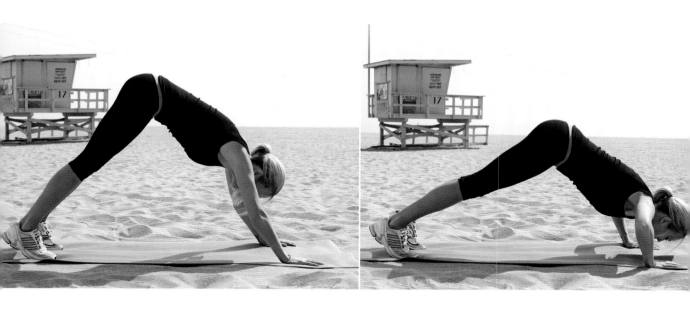

SHOULDER PRESS IN YOGA POSE

On all fours, come into the downward-facing dog yoga pose. Lift your heels so that you're standing on your toes. Bring down your upper body by pressing your elbows outward, placing your head in between your hands. Imagine your head coming an inch or two lower with each press. Perform twelve presses.

Tip!

Since you have less fat on your arms and shoulders, you'll get visible results from your workout in no time!

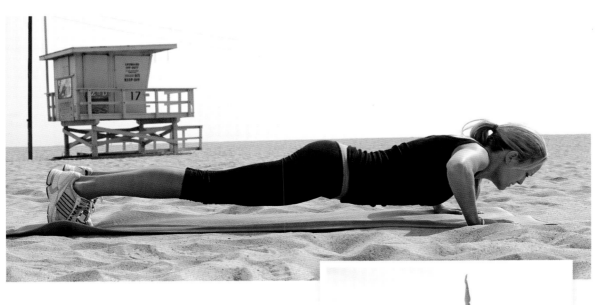

T PUSH-UP

Push-ups with a twist are one of the easiest and best bodyweight exercises to improve the muscles in your chest, arms, shoulders, and core.

Come into the push-up position and lower your body, as in a normal push-up. When you come back up, put all your weight on your left arm as you turn your right side upward, extending your right hand straight above your head. Return to the starting position, perform another push-up, and come up again, extending the left arm. Repeat three times on each side, being sure to keep your core tight, for a total of six T push-ups.

Tip!
Make this exercise easier by bending your knees for the push-up.

6

SIDE TRICEPS PUSH-UP

This exercise activates your triceps, eliminates wobbling, and targets the biceps muscles. Your obliques will get a workout, too.

Lie on your left side with bent knees, hugging your waist with your left arm. Place your right palm on the mat in front of you. Press yourself up to a sort of side sit-up with the help of your right arm. If you can, lift your feet from the mat as well. Come down again and perform twelve repetitions on each side for a total of twenty-four.

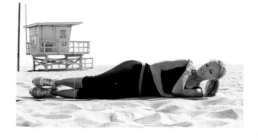

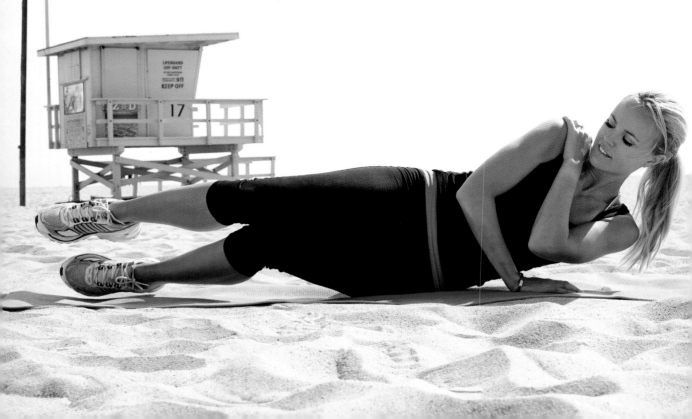

ARMS/SHOULDERS OVERVIEW»

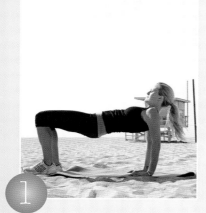

TRICEPS DIPS *x 12*

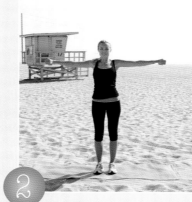

SHOULDER FLY *x 30*

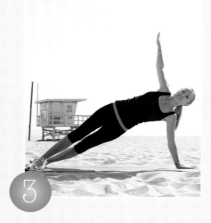

PLANK WITH DUMBBELL ROWS *x 12*

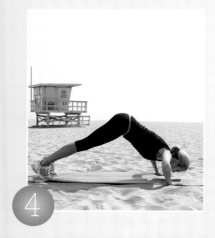

SHOULDER PRESS IN YOGA POSE *x 12*

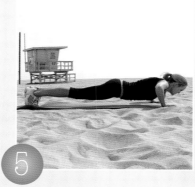

T PUSH-UP *x 6*

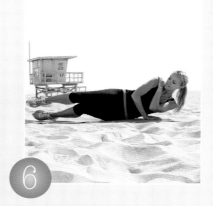

SIDE TRICEPS PUSH-UP *x 24*

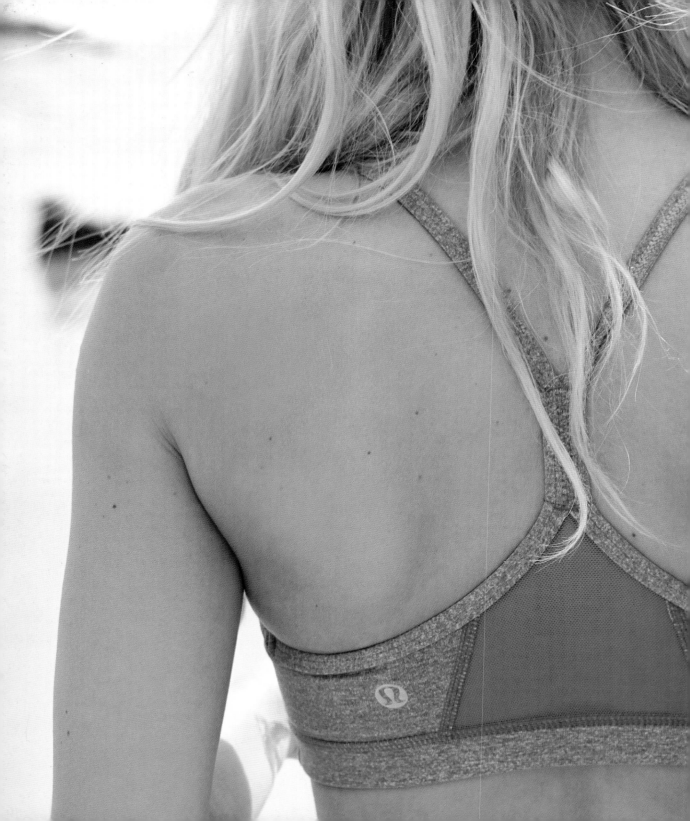

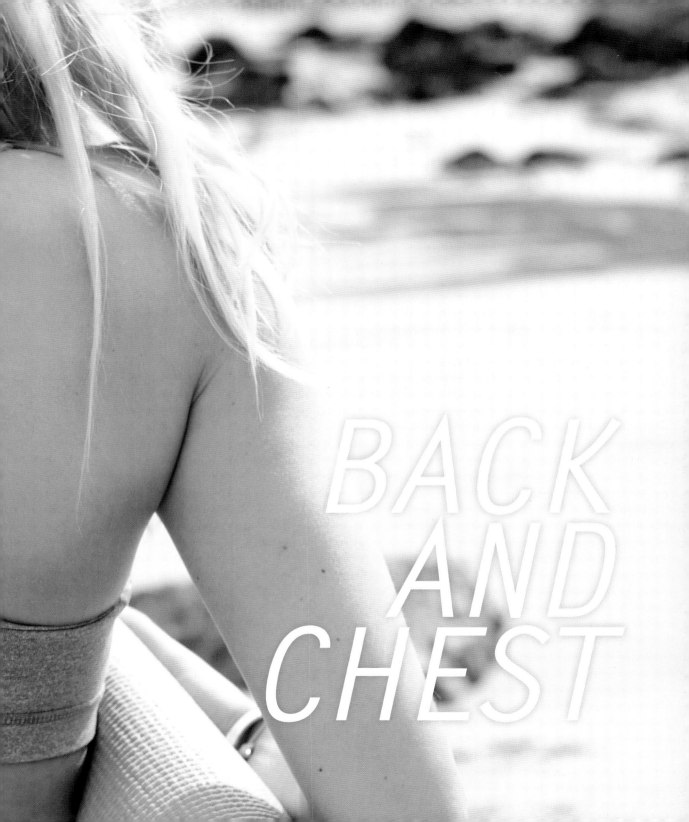

BACK AND CHEST

BACK AND CHEST»

If there's one thing I have problems with, it's my posture. I sit hunched over like a cheese puff at my computer every day, and I stretch about as often as leap years come. I should add that I think back workouts are among the most boring things around. But training your back is an investment in the future. I've learned that from all the trainers I've met. Obviously, I'd like to avoid problems with my back, turning into the next Quasimodo, that sort of thing.

When I asked model trainer Joe Dowdell at Peak Performance Gym in New York, "What are your best tips to look fit?" his reply was "Good posture."

If you have strong back and chest muscles (and yes, you need to train both), you'll give a more fit impression. You'll also feel more self-confident and secure when you have proud, straight posture!

I try to remind myself every day to stretch, but that's not enough; I've got to do proper workouts, too. So I do these exercises, which help me to build up strength. Let's go!

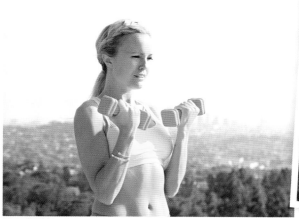
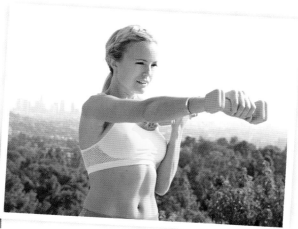
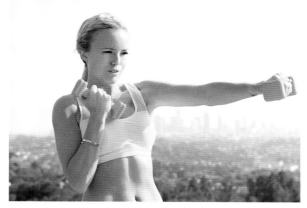

Tip! Make this exercise more challenging by scissor-jumping as you box.

WEIGHT BOXING

Stand upright with your feet shoulder width apart, your knees slightly bent. Hold two light dumbbells or water bottles in your hands. Lift both arms as in a biceps curl. When your elbows are bent, turn your right hand so that the palm faces your chest. Now bring the arm out and forward, turning your palm toward the ground as in a straight boxing punch. Bring your arm back and alternate both arms, standing and "boxing" for one minute. Rest for ten seconds, then continue for one more minute without a break.

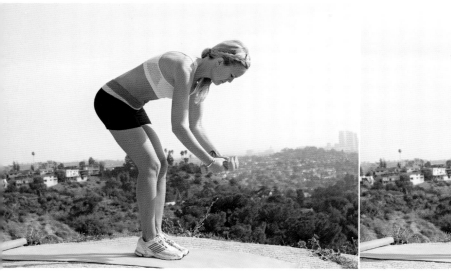
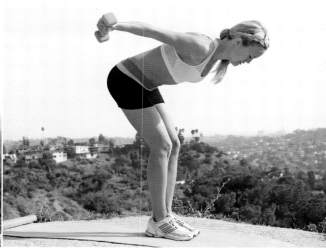

FLAT-BACK FLY

Stand with your legs shoulder width apart, a
dumbbell or water bottle in each hand. Lower
your upper body from your hips, keeping your
back straight. Begin with your hands under your
chest and bring them straight out to the side like
a bird's wings, feeling how the shoulder blades
really pinch together as you bring your arms out.
Remain in this position and perform fifteen flyes.

3

DIAGONAL

Start on all fours on a soft surface. Keep your back as straight as possible with your hands directly under your shoulders. Lift one arm and the opposite leg, stretching them out as far as possible; remain in this position for three seconds before returning to the starting position and repeating the exercise. Perform twelve lifts on each side for a total of twenty-four.

Tip! This exercise stabilizes both your hips and core while strengthening your back and improving your posture.

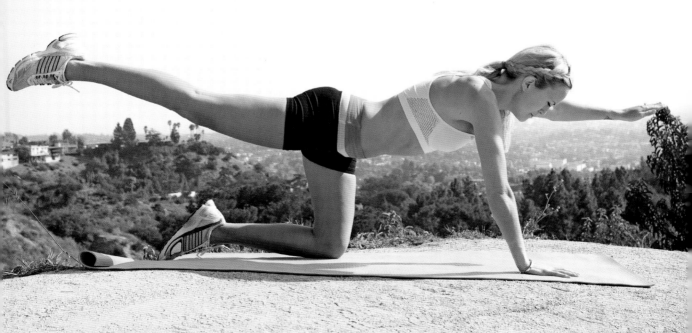

SUPERWOMAN

Lie on your stomach with your arms at your sides, palms facing down. Tighten the muscles in your booty and lower back, lifting your upper body and legs from the ground at the same time. Turn your arms up at the same time so your palms face upward. Keep your neck straight and hold this position for a few seconds before returning to the starting position. Repeat twelve times.

Tip!
This exercise strengthens your lower back most of all, which is good if you spend a lot of time sitting at your computer. The gluteus maximus, the largest muscle in your booty, also gets a workout.

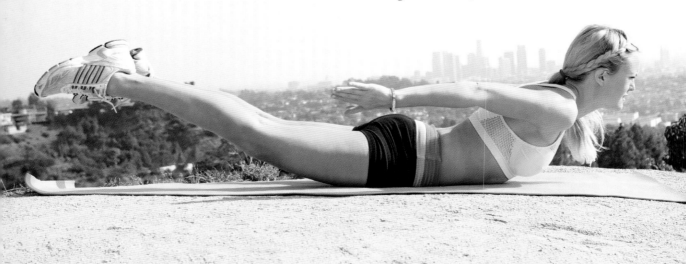

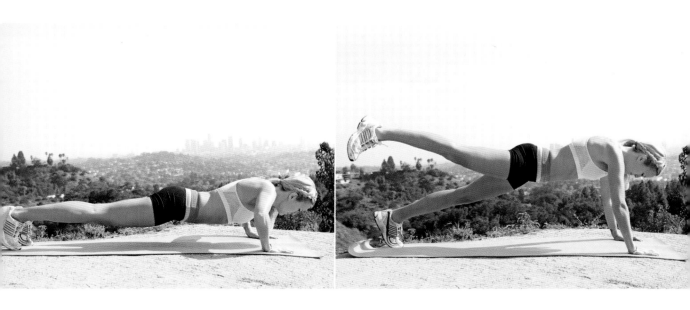

PUSH-UP WITH LEG RAISE

Come into the kneeling push-up position, so you have a straight line from your shoulders down to your ankles. Bend your elbows and lower yourself into a push-up. Press yourself back up while lifting your right foot behind you about an inch off the floor. Release the foot back down. For an easier variation, perform the push-ups on your knees instead. Remember to come up for the leg lift, though. Perform twelve push-ups with lifts, alternating legs.

Y-T-I

Together, these three movements help to strengthen the muscles in your upper back and shoulders. It's the perfect exercise for dresses with deep backs.

Lie on your stomach, bringing your gaze to the floor in front of you. Bring your arms above your head, forming a Y; then bring them out to the sides to make a T; finally, bring them straight out in front of you, making an I with your body. Repeat these Y-T-I movements twelve times without a break.

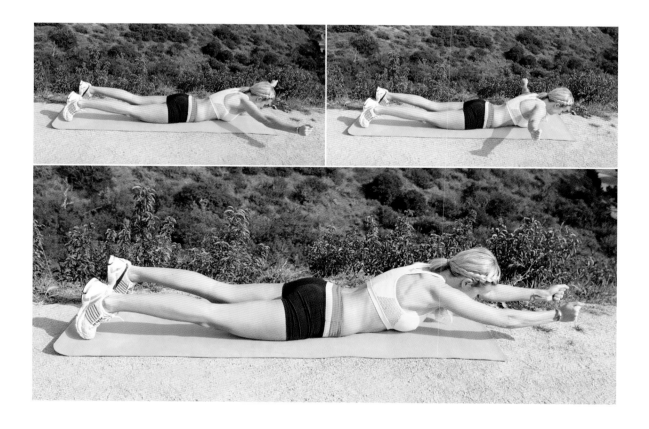

BACK/CHEST OVERVIEW

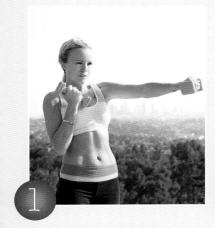

1 WEIGHT BOXING *2 MIN*

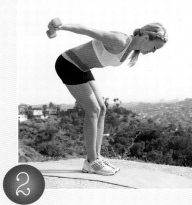

2 FLAT-BACK FLY *X 15*

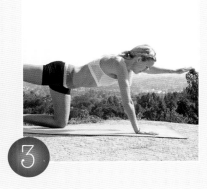

3 DIAGONAL *X 24*

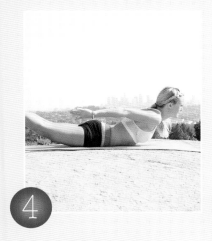

4 SUPERWOMAN *X 12*

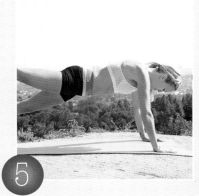

5 PUSH-UP WITH LEG RAISE *X 12*

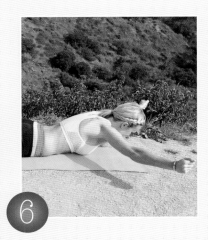

6 Y-T-I *X 12*

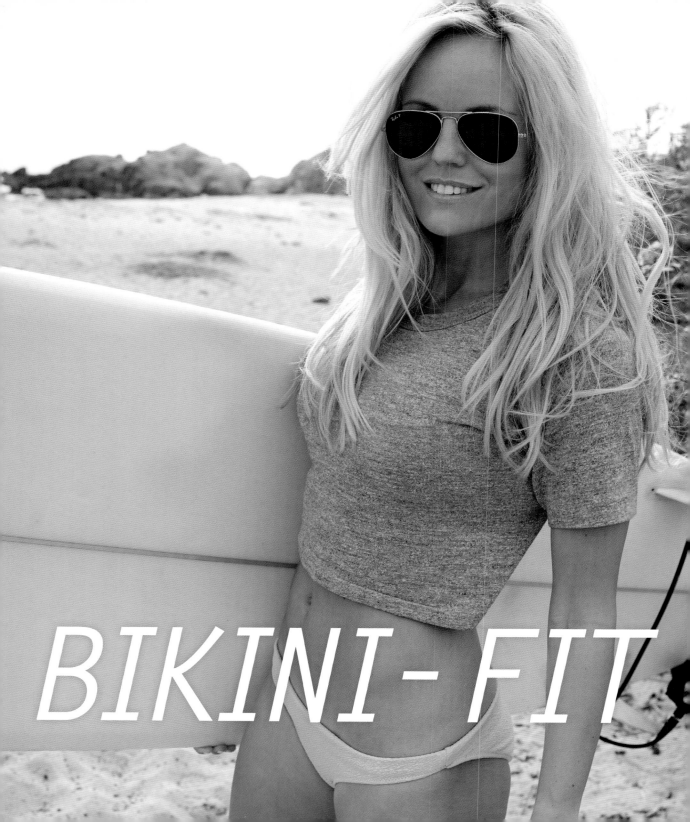

BIKINI - FIT

Burn calories and tone up fast!

Sometimes—OK, often—I want to get things done fast! If you're like me and hardly have time to wait for nail polish to dry, I've got a workout for you. You don't need to spend hours running or in the gym. Studies show that explosive exercises where you challenge your whole body, your heart, and your strength are the absolute most effective ones for burning calories and toning up—fast!

With this explosive and super-intense whole body workout, you'll challenge your muscle tone and strength, whipping your pulse up to the max. The result? You'll burn more calories in a shorter time, even after your workout is over.

Fifteen minutes is completely manageable if you perform all the exercises as explosively as possible. Yes, that means you need to fly when you jump, and come down into some deeeep squats—your thighs should be burning! Your body gets a good challenge and things really happen when you push yourself outside of your comfort zone. And best of all: you can do this workout outside, in the sun, without any equipment whatsoever.

Get ready to see some results!

«BIKINI-FIT IN FIFTEEN MINUTES

1

BURPEES

I'll be honest. This exercise is absolutely vile—but it's also insanely effective. You might not ever come to love burpees, but you'll love the results you get doing them! This exercise challenges all the muscles in your body and is a fiendishly effective fat burner. Feel the burn!

Start in a push-up position with your weight evenly distributed between your hands and toes. Jump your feet up to your hands, coming up in an explosive jump with your hands held high. Try to land softly on both feet, then come back down to the starting position. Repeat the exercise without pausing after landings. Perform ten to twelve burpees.

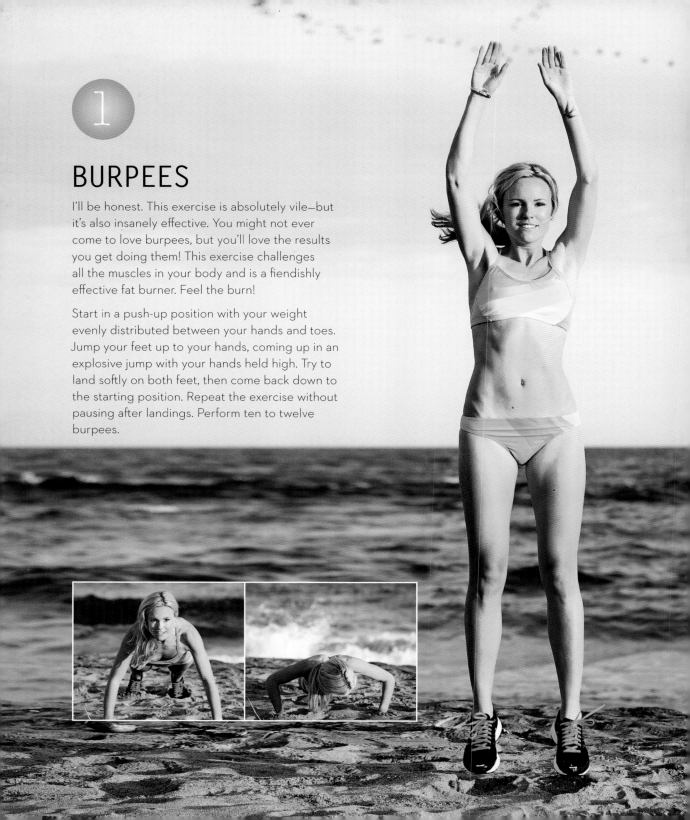

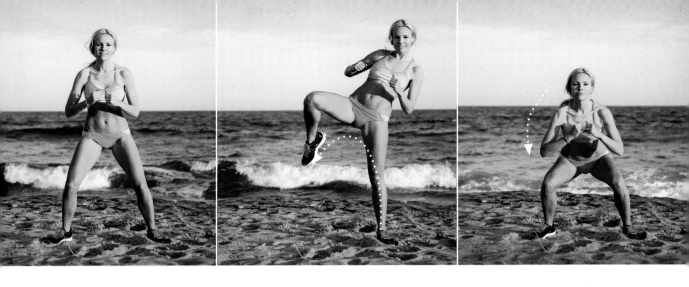

SUMO KICK

This exercise helps to slim down those stubborn fat deposits on your inner and outer thighs while toning the area where your bikini meets your booty. Anything loose gets tightened right up!

Stand with your feet wide, hands on your hips.

Lift your right leg from the knee, rotating it to the side in a sort of half-moon. Set the foot down and come down into a medium-depth squat, channeling your inner sumo wrestler. When you come up from the squat, lift your right leg again and kick it out with the heel to the side, as if to kick an opponent in a kickboxing match. Repeat with the left leg. Perform twenty-four kicks, twelve with each leg.

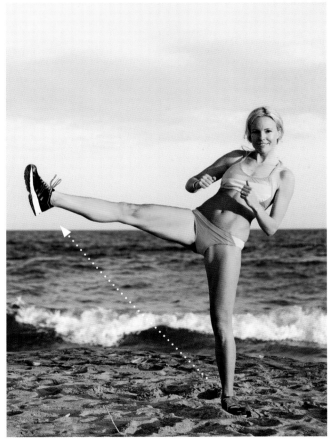

EXPLOSIVE LUNGE JUMP

Lunges are the most effective exercise for sculpting your legs, thighs, and a round aerobics booty.

Take a big step forward with your right leg so your left knee nearly touches the ground. Stand like a skier in this lunge position before jumping straight up and switching your leg position, bringing your left leg in front of your right leg. Continue jumping and switching the leg in front as you hold yourself in as low a position as possible.

Perform twenty jumps, then rest for ten seconds and perform twenty more.

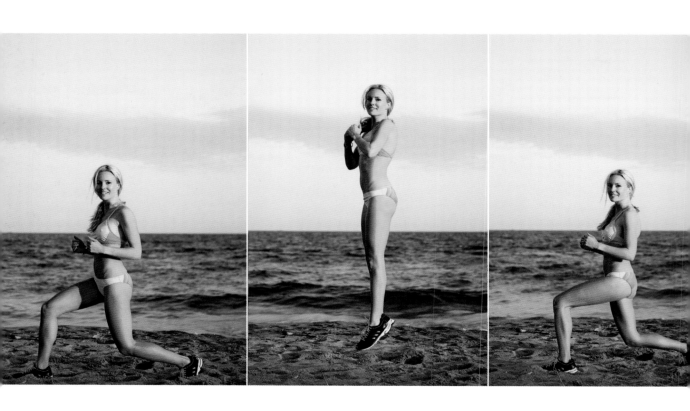

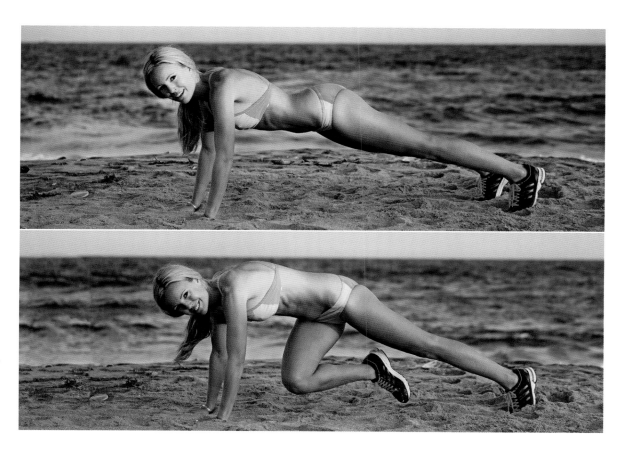

MOUNTAIN CLIMBER

You'll work your entire body here, especially your arms and core.

Come into the plank position with straight arms. Tighten your core and lower your booty, then bring your right knee in toward your stomach. Bring it back with control and continue by bringing your left leg in toward your stomach, being sure not to lift your booty too much or lose the strong posture in your core. Perform twenty-five mountain climbers.

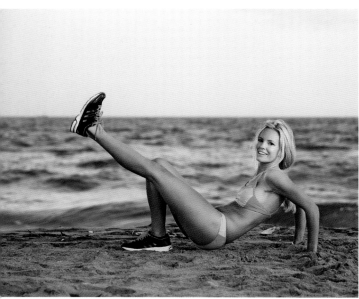 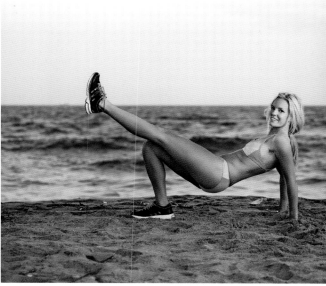

TRICEPS DIPS

Sit on the ground with your knees bent, feet a short distance in front of you. Place your hands on the ground with your fingers facing forward. Press yourself upward so you stand like a table. Keeping a steady position, bend your arms until your elbows reach a 90-degree angle while lifting your right leg and stretching it straight out in front of you. Press up to the straight-arm position once more as you release the leg back down. Perform another dip, this time stretching out the left leg before returning to the table position. Perform six lifts with each leg for a total of twelve dips. Rest, then perform twelve more.

Tip!

This exercise quickly adds definition to your arm muscles, since it slims and sculpts the shoulders and the backs of the upper arms.

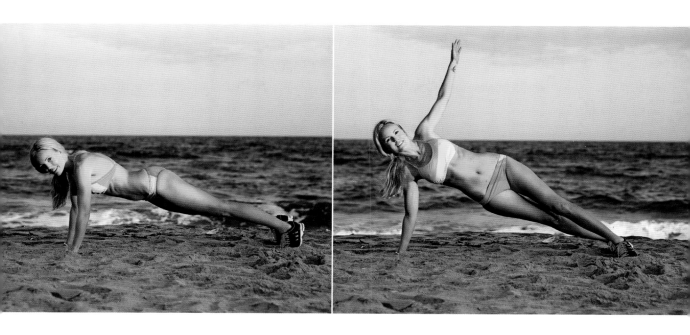

T PUSH-UPS

Push-ups with a twist are some of the easiest and best bodyweight exercises to improve the muscles in your chest, arms, shoulders, and core.

Come into a push-up position, lowering your body as in a normal push-up. When you come back up, place all your weight on your left arm while turning your right side up and stretching out your right hand directly above your head. Return to the starting position, perform another push-up, and now stretch out the left arm. Perform three T push-ups on each side, being sure to keep your core tight the whole time.

Tip!
Remember: the more you sweat, the heavier you breathe, and the tougher you train, the more you burn!

TRICKS TO STICK TO YOUR WORKOUT PLAN

1 YOU SNOOZE, YOU LOSE

This is one of Sofi's favorite quotes! So kick your snoozing habit, get up, and get active! The morning usually sets the tone for the whole day, so by starting off great you're set to have an awesome day. It might be as easy as waking up thirty minutes earlier so you can enjoy a nice long breakfast or a morning run before work. Or maybe some quality time with your boyfriend or husband! Also remember to stay positive; one small positive thought in the morning can change your whole day.

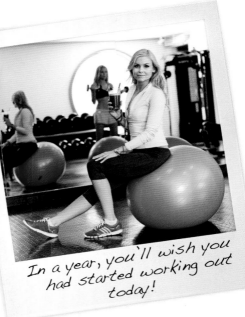

In a year, you'll wish you had started working out today!

2 TRAIN WITH A BUDDY

You won't always be excited for your workout, but if you work out with a buddy, it'll be harder to cancel your jog in favor of a Project Runway marathon on the sofa. We love to run together or take power walks. It's a perfect way to socialize and get your workout done at the same time.

3 DEVELOP A GOOD TARGET IMAGE

You often hear talk of two kinds of motivation: internal and external. External motivation, like seeing yourself in a sexy bikini, can be a good kick-start, but internal motivation, based on your health, is what'll really keep you going until you reach your goal.

If your outlook is focused on your health, like wanting more energy during the day, better sleep, or simply feeling better overall, you'll automatically have a stronger motivational base that will always give you a reason to train.

4 BE FLEXIBLE

Did you have to work late? Again?

Don't see unexpected obstacles on the way as new reasons to put off working out. Forget that all-or-nothing mind-set. It's not individual moments but what you do most of the time that matters in the long run. Be flexible. Just because you had to work late and missed your planned gym class, you can still go for a walk or a short run later. Be flexible!

5 PEPPY PLAYLIST

It's been shown that upbeat, energetic music can boost your motivation and endurance. Don't believe us? Take our top ten power-pep tracks for a spin. We guarantee they'll have you Beyoncé-strutting your way to your workout!

JULIA'S TOP-10-POWER-PEP-TRACKS

1. Run the World (Girls) – Beyoncé
2. Leave the World Behind – David Guetta
3. Firework – Katy Perry
4. I Made It – Kevin Rudolf (ft. Birdman, Jay Sean & Lil Wayne)
5. When I Grow Up – Pussycat Dolls
6. Best of You – Foo Fighters
7. Since U Been Gone – Kelly Clarkson
8. Work it Out – Lil Jon (ft. Pitbull)
9. Stronger – Kanye West
10. Don't Stop Believin' – Journey

SOFI'S TOP-10-POWER-PEP-TRACKS

1. Eye of the Tiger – Survivor
2. Wild Ones – Flo Rida
3. Beautiful People – Chris Brown (ft. Benny Benassi)
4. Marry the Night – Lady Gaga
5. I'm Sexy and I Know It – LMFAO
6. Moves Like Jagger – Maroon 5 (ft. Christina Aguilera)
7. Run the World – Beyoncé
8. Movin' Too Fast – Artful Dodger
9. World Hold On – Bob Sinclar
10. Beat It – Michael Jackson

6 SET YOUR CLOTHES OUT

Set out your workout clothing near your bed before going to sleep. When your alarm rings in the morning, all you've got to do is put them on and you're ready to go. Do it right away, without even thinking! As soon as you start watching

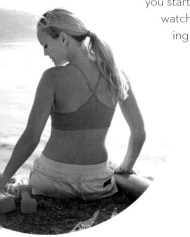

morning TV shows and checking your email, it's all too easy to get stuck doing that instead.

7 MEASURE YOUR RESULTS

Kick out the scale! Don't let it be the one thing that decides whether you're making progress. Fat and muscle have the same mass but a different density, so even if you don't see any change on the scale, your body is making progress. Throw out the scale and measure the way your clothes fit, how great you feel when you wake up, and how much energy you have in everyday life. That's what really matters!

8 READ MAGAZINES OR BLOGS

Read a fitness magazine while you have lunch and there's a good chance you'll also be hungry for that before-dinner workout you were thinking about skipping. Looking at or thinking about someone you admire for his or her healthy choices will make you more inclined to follow his or her example.

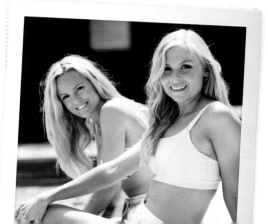

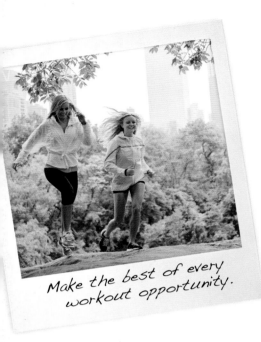

Make the best of every workout opportunity.

10 GET OUT OF THE DOLDRUMS

You're not the only one fighting against shaky motivation. Even the most strongly motivated people have their ups and downs. If you're not feeling it right now, know that it'll come back. Until it does, just don't give up. Try to bring back what inspired you in the beginning. Test out new exercise classes and give yourself permission to do light workouts. What's important is that you keep going.

9 BE ACTIVE EVERY DAY

Don't feel bad if you don't have the time to go to the gym every other day. You don't have to! Being active is so much more important. The main secret to more energy and a healthier lifestyle is to get active on a daily basis—for example, by walking everywhere, taking the stairs, or playing with your kids. Every time you move your body, your brain releases natural pleasure-producing chemicals such as endorphins and dopamine. It's the easiest and best way to feel better instantly.

11 WORKING OUT—YOUR LUXURY TIME

Does your workout feel like a chore or a punishment? It's certainly not something you look forward to. Turn your mind-set around, though, and see your workout as a slice of "you time" where you can reward your body and make it sexier, stronger, and healthier. Feel that you're doing something good for yourself and that you and your body are a team working together. When you start to pep yourself up and see your workout as an opportunity to show your body gratitude and appreciation, it'll make an incredible difference.

12 NO EXCUSES

Do you try to find excuses to skip your workout? Stop sabotaging yourself. If you're the kind of girl who always puts things off until tomorrow, next Monday, or after Easter, you're never going to see any changes. To borrow an old but very good slogan from a certain brand of sporting goods: just do it!

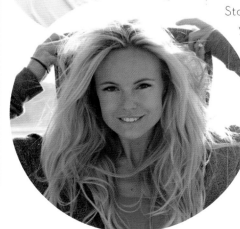

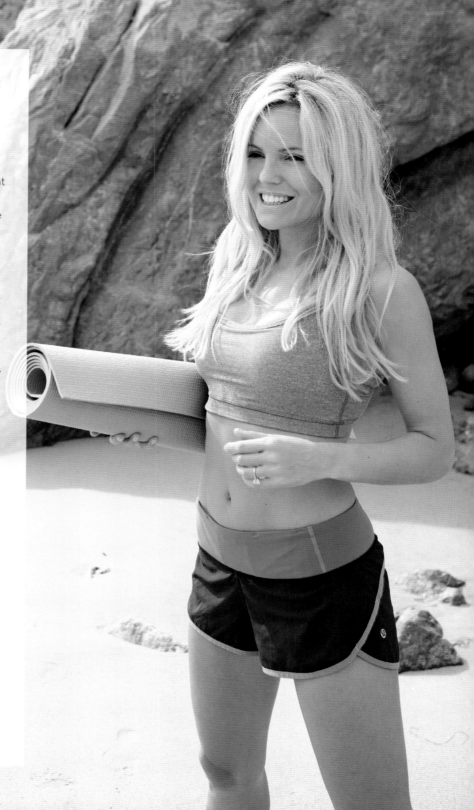

13 TAKE IT ONE DAY AT A TIME

Sometimes big goals can feel overwhelming. So instead of focusing on all of the hours of sweat standing between you and your goal, just take it one day at a time and focus on what's right in front of you, here and now. An hour's workout doesn't sound so bad today, don't you think?

14 SHARE

Blog, tweet, Facebook! If you keep your goals to yourself, perhaps you're secretly afraid to be held accountable and really make those changes. After all, once you've said it, you've got to do it, too!

15 REWARD YOURSELF

This one's our favorite! Reward yourself as you reach small goals along the way, like being able to run a whole lap without walking part of the way, or doing all your workouts this week. Treat yourself to something that's not associated with sweets or other unhealthy stuff. A massage, a new piece of clothing, some lovely nail polish, or a glossy fashion magazine all make perfect presents for yourself.

BEST PT-TIPS

They train some of the world's most heavily guarded and coveted bodies. Naturally, they must have some exceptional tips to share! During our travels and interviews for Sofi's Mode throughout the years, we've collected the best tips from the world's best personal trainers.

WEAR COMFY SHOES!

GET yourself a pair of real comfy athletic shoes so you can start walking everywhere. Everyday activity is undervalued and really makes an enormous difference.

LOOK at your workout as an everyday task. It should be as natural a part of your life as brushing your teeth or eating breakfast. Try to train every day, even if it's only for a short while. My clients often don't exercise for more than twenty-five minutes at a time, but they do it every day, and that's what gives results.

SHORTEN your resting time when doing strength training by pausing for twenty to thirty seconds between each exercise. That way, you can maximize your training time in the gym and shorten your workout by up to 20 percent.

DON'T slack off just because you're on vacation; with a pair of athletic shoes, a resistance band, and a workout DVD, you can easily work out in your hotel room.

DON´T WORK OUT HARDER, WORK OUT SMARTER.

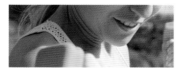

YOUR OWN BODY WEIGHT IS YOUR BEST GYM.

ABOVE ALL, there are no shortcuts. Everyone wants to know if there's a quick fix—there's not. Getting off your booty and taking charge of your fitness is the only thing that works.

SET aside time to integrate yoga or Pilates into your workout routine; it relaxes you and reduces your cortisol levels.

DON'T be afraid to gain weight. Putting on muscle mass will only give your body sexy curves.

WORK OUT IN THE MORNING AND FILL YOUR DAY WITH HEAPS OF ENERGY!

MORNINGS are the best time to work out since you'll be filled with energy that lasts all day and motivates you to make good choices. Physiologically, your body will also burn more fat before getting calories from breakfast.

LUNGES are the absolute best exercise for your booty and thighs, especially if you combine them with kicks and jumps.

ONE of the most important things I tell my clients is to really think about the training they're doing. If you want to train your booty, your thoughts should be focused on your booty. It sounds kind of funny, but by focusing all your mental energy on the region you're working on, you'll get better results.

FIND A WORKOUT THAT YOU TRULY ENJOY; YOU WILL NATURALLY DO MORE OF WHAT MAKES YOU HAPPY.

FIND a fitness program based on how you want to look. If you don't want to look like a bodybuilder, don't pick a male personal trainer who looks like one. Don't fuss over it, either; the less equipment you need, the better.

WHATEVER you're training, see to it that you can wring sweat out of your top when you're finished. People don't understand how important it is to really sweat and give it your all. If you still look cute after your workout, you haven't worked out hard enough.

MAKE EVERY WORKOUT COUNT; ONLY YOU CAN MAKE IT HAPPEN!

ANY sort of aerobic activity is good if you want to lose weight. Running, rowing, and cycling are all good choices. But if you want to sculpt your body and shape your booty and thighs, it's strength training with weights that'll give you what you want. That's how you get visible results.

THE best exercise is whatever you do naturally! Do you enjoy running but find cycling dull? Run! When all is said and done, the exercise you actually do is what gives you results.

JUMP, JUMP! A JUMP-ROPE IS ALL YOU NEED FOR A GOOD CARDIO WORKOUT.

GET out your jump-rope! Jumping rope is one of the most effective exercises to work your entire body, and it can burn up to two hundred calories in just fifteen minutes.

WIND down and reduce stress with some sit-ups before you go to sleep. Just five minutes- worth of exercise will actually improve your sleep quality.

MAKE sure you get enough vitamin D. It's one of the most important factors of optimal health and is vital for your nervous system, immune system, and the burning of fat.

"IF YOU LOOK CUTE AFTER YOUR WORK-OUT, YOU HAVEN'T TRAINED HARD ENOUGH!"

TRACY ANDERSON

Tone Up That Tummy!

Stress, PMS, and the wrong kind of diet can make your tummy protest—in a big way! You probably know that feeling you get after a long flight, or when you wake up after a weekend of partying and discover that your stomach looks a bit on the pregnant side. This bloating comes from your body collecting excessive amounts of water, which can happen because of hormonal changes when you're about to begin, or have just finished, your menstrual cycle; when you've eaten a lot of extra carbohydrates and salt, which bind liquids; or when you've been traveling by air. As luck would have it, there are tips to help you quickly get rid of this bloating.

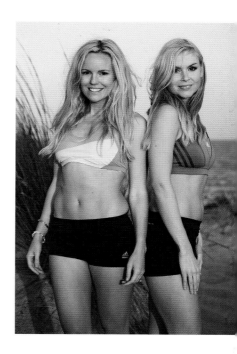

Your stomach often feels bloated

Constantly walking around feeling bloated is a sign that something's wrong. Take a look at your diet. Perhaps you're lactose- or gluten-intolerant? Try replacing normal dairy products with lactose-free ones for a couple of weeks and cut out wheat, corn, and rye from your diet. Don't forget to eat five small meals a day, either, and try to reduce stress. When you start to eat regularly and increase your protein intake, the problem will often disappear on its own. Also try taking probiotic tablets, which you can find at the pharmacy.

You become bloated before or during your menstrual cycle

Unfortunately, bloating is often one of the less fun parts of being a woman. But don't feel unmotivated and down just because you're bloated for a few days of the month—hang in there! Soon, your body will naturally return to its normal self. Until then, treat yourself to a little dark chocolate and a banana or two. Bananas contain potassium, which flushes salt—which can cause you to retain too much water—out of your body.

You're going on a hot date

A bloated stomach and a tight dress are no dream combination. The best you can do to get rid of the excess liquid quickly is actually to cleanse your body with even more liquid. Too little water will cause your body to retain more of it, so try to drink six to eight cups a day. Water speeds up your metabolism and jump-starts a sluggish stomach, which can often be one of the reasons for bloating. Take a short walk. As little as ten minutes of walking can relieve bloating by bringing up your metabolism and causing your bowels to work faster. If this fails, Spanx is your friend (slimming underwear—Google it!)!

You're headed out for a sunny vacation

Focus on eating great, natural, and healthy foods before your trip so you don't upset your tummy. Probiotics, which can be found in yogurt, are great for calming an upset stomach when you travel. Also remember that confidence is your best outfit, especially on the beach. Rock it and own it!

The worst stomach saboteurs

ALCOHOL: Not only will it make you hunger for fatty, salty foods but people who drink more than a glass a day have been shown to be thicker around their stomachs than people who stick to one glass or less.

STRESS: When you're stressed or worried for longer periods of time, your body releases the hormone cortisol, which causes you to store more fat around your stomach. Take a look at your lifestyle and see what you can change.

CARBONATED DRINKS: Too many bubbles in your mineral water can result in an excess of gases in your stomach.

SALT: It can take up to three days for your body to eliminate all the water your body has collected after excessive salt intake. Just like sugar, unfortunately, large amounts of salt tend to hide in restaurant food and processed foods, as well as in bread and cottage cheese. Learn to season your food with other flavorings besides salt, such as freshly squeezed lemon juice.

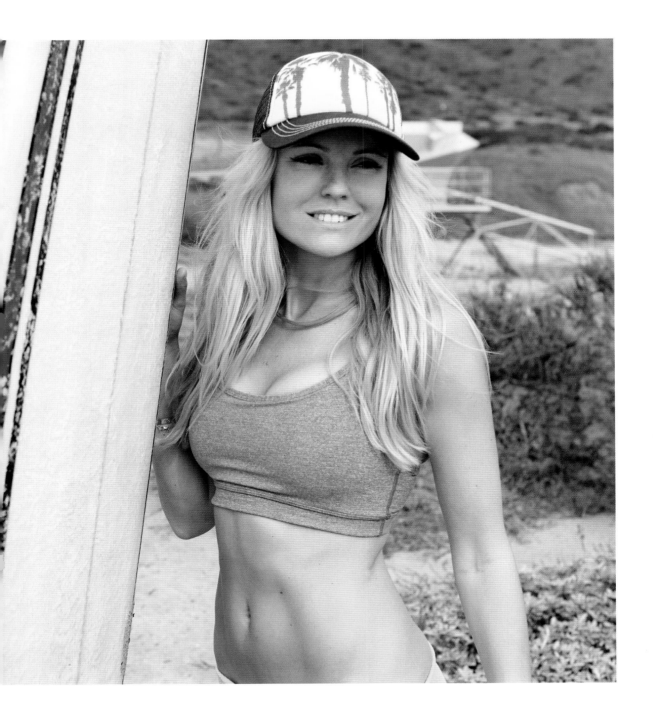

WHITE BREAD, POTATOES, AND SUGAR: Foods that raise your blood sugar can quickly turn into fat around your tummy. Potatoes are the worst, as they've shown themselves to have an especially high tendency to be stored as stomach fat.

PRODUCTS WITH SWEETENERS: Chewing gum, throat lozenges, and other products that contain xylitol and sorbitol are other items to avoid. These items greatly increase the buildup of gas.

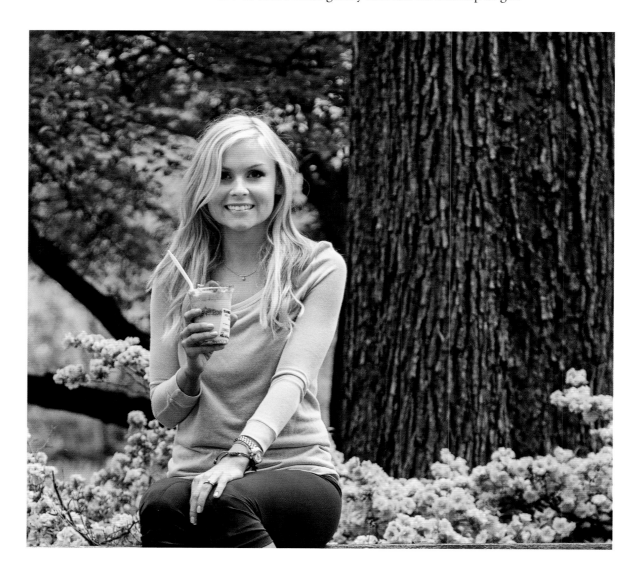

MAXIMIZE YOUR WORKOUT WITH THE RIGHT FOOD

How you're feeling on any given day isn't the only thing that determines how much energy you'll have for your workout. The food you eat both before and after can actually improve your performance, fat burning, muscle growth, and recovery. So put a little extra energy into eating right, and you'll get twice as much back.

Before your workout—give your body a Bodylicious boost

Lots of girls think it's smart to work out on an empty stomach. But unless we're talking about a low-intensity walk in the morning, that's actually not a good idea at all. The less you eat, the more your body works to retain fat. If you're going to do any exercise more intense than walking, you should always eat, both before and after your workout. Studies show that you burn more fat and experience faster muscle growth if you eat both before and after your workout.

A piece of fruit before your workout isn't enough

You need something that contains both proteins and carbohydrates, but less fat and fiber. Fat takes longer to break down, and when you're training, you want to avoid reducing the flow of blood to your muscles. Eating a bit of candy or sweets right before a workout might seem like a smart idea—after all, you're going to burn all those calories anyway. Unfortunately, it doesn't work quite like that in practice. Foods with a high glycemic index increase your body's insulin levels, which works against your body's ability to burn fat. On the other hand, you can eat a piece of chocolate or something else sweet right after your workout in good conscience. Your metabolism will be at its peak then, and your body will use that sugar instead of storing it as fat.

Bodylicious workout boost meals:

- A bowl of yogurt with berries and müsli
- A banana and ⅓ cup of cottage cheese with cinnamon
- Fruit salad with a dollop of ricotta or cottage cheese, and 5 chopped walnuts
- A slice of whole-wheat bread with egg, turkey, and tomato
- ¾ cup shrimp with an egg and ¼ of an avocado

GO BANANAS! NATURE'S OWN ENERGY BAR, A BANANA, IS PERFECT FOR INSTANT ENERGY AND RECOVERY.

Add a little extra energy by eating right.

BODYLICIOUS !
tip !

The one exception: working out before breakfast

If you want to boost your fat-burning by taking walks in the mornings, you can wait until after to eat. Since morning walks are low-intensity exercise, you'll burn more fat if your body doesn't need to draw from the food first. Have a glass of water and a cup of coffee before you head out. Besides the alertness you get from the coffee, caffeine encourages the release of fat from fat cells. One or two cups in the morning before training has been shown to improve muscle strength, concentration, and performance while working out.

Time for your After Workout!

You can't afford to miss this after workout! During your workout, your body consumes the carbohydrates stored in your muscles, while simultaneously breaking down the muscles, to a certain degree. That's why it's extra important to fill up on protein and carbohydrates after your workout so you can build up your body again. The first forty-five minutes after you finish your workout, your muscles act like sponges, sucking in and absorbing all the nutrients they can get. So don't wait until you get home to eat if you have a long route to get there; instead, make sure you bring something to eat in your bag. By having a recovery meal immediately after your workout, you can store a greater amount of glycogen in your muscles than you'd be able to if you waited more than an hour since finishing your training. And if you wait even longer than that, it can take up to three or four days before you've completely recovered from your workout.

Bodylicious recovery meals

- Eggs, in all forms: in omelettes, scrambled, on a sandwich . . . An egg, depending on its size, contains six to eight grams of protein.
- Light cottage cheese with berries or chopped fruit and some nuts. A tub of cottage cheese contains a whole 32.5 grams of protein.
- A smoothie with light yogurt, berries, banana, and müsli.

Protein shake

Are you in a hurry after your workout? Do you find that you can hardly wait until the next large meal? If so, a protein shake is the best way for you to recover quickly. Both whey and soy protein powders contain about the same amount of protein, about twenty to thirty grams a scoop. We prefer whey protein, since it's taken up quickly by muscles and has been shown to stimulate their recovery faster than soy protein. One of our favorite proteins is from Herbalife. What's most important is that the powder doesn't have any added sugar and contains minimal carbohydrates. Buy a stainless steel thermos and prepare your shake in the morning.

BODYLICIOUS SHAPE-UP SMOOTHIE

- 1 ¾ cups (414 mL) reduced/low fat or almond milk
- 1 scoop vanilla- or berry-flavored protein powder
- ½ banana
- 1 handful strawberries (frozen or fresh)

Our smoothie contains both muscle-building protein and the right amount of carbohydrates to keep up your muscles' glycogen reserves—your energy when you're working out! Mix all the ingredients in a blender and top with ice. Drink immediately or pour into a stainless steel thermos, so it'll stay cold, and take it to the gym.

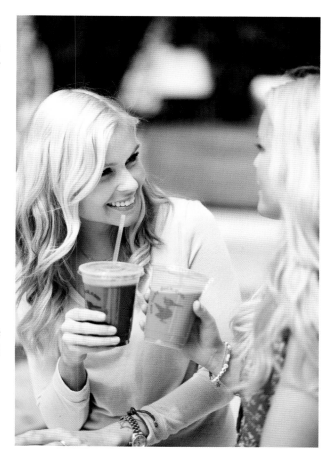

Will I have a bigger appetite from exercising more?

No, getting hungrier as a result of regular exercise is actually a myth. Many who begin exercising more intensely simultaneously increase their food intake because they feel that they need to eat more. But slamming down giant portions isn't actually necessary unless you've been doing some extremely intense workouts. Most often, eating normally is enough; just add in a recovery meal or an extra protein shake.

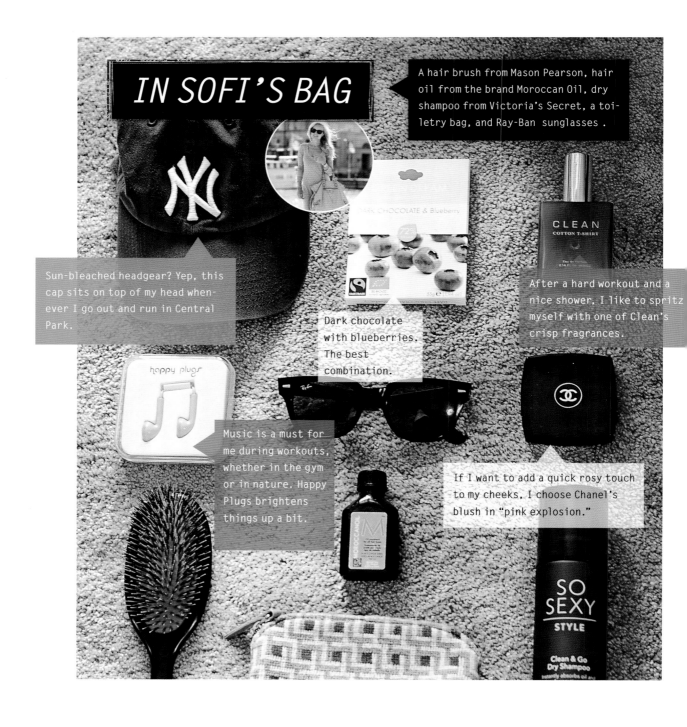

IN SOFI'S BAG

A hair brush from Mason Pearson, hair oil from the brand Moroccan Oil, dry shampoo from Victoria's Secret, a toiletry bag, and Ray-Ban sunglasses.

Sun-bleached headgear? Yep, this cap sits on top of my head whenever I go out and run in Central Park.

Dark chocolate with blueberries. The best combination.

After a hard workout and a nice shower, I like to spritz myself with one of Clean's crisp fragrances.

Music is a must for me during workouts, whether in the gym or in nature. Happy Plugs brightens things up a bit.

If I want to add a quick rosy touch to my cheeks, I choose Chanel's blush in "pink explosion."

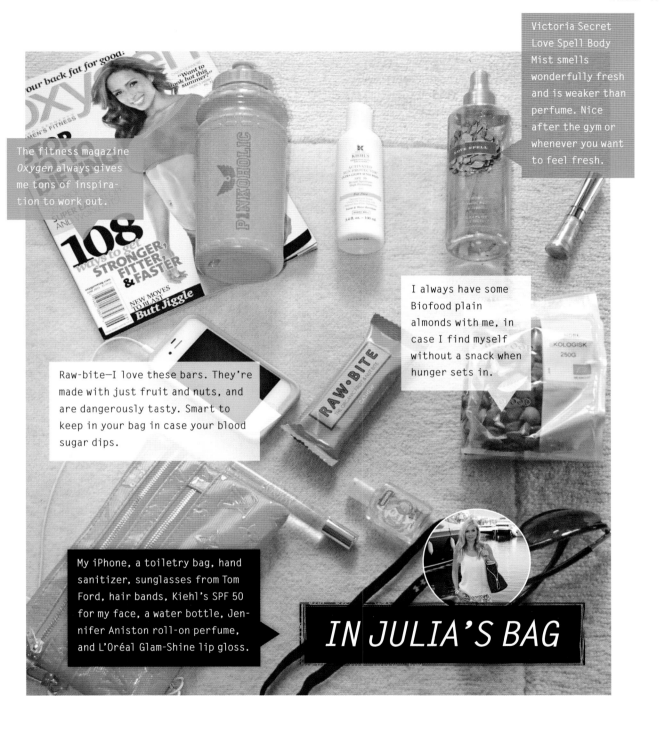

Victoria Secret Love Spell Body Mist smells wonderfully fresh and is weaker than perfume. Nice after the gym or whenever you want to feel fresh.

The fitness magazine *Oxygen* always gives me tons of inspiration to work out.

I always have some Biofood plain almonds with me, in case I find myself without a snack when hunger sets in.

Raw-bite—I love these bars. They're made with just fruit and nuts, and are dangerously tasty. Smart to keep in your bag in case your blood sugar dips.

My iPhone, a toiletry bag, hand sanitizer, sunglasses from Tom Ford, hair bands, Kiehl's SPF 50 for my face, a water bottle, Jennifer Aniston roll-on perfume, and L'Oréal Glam-Shine lip gloss.

IN JULIA'S BAG

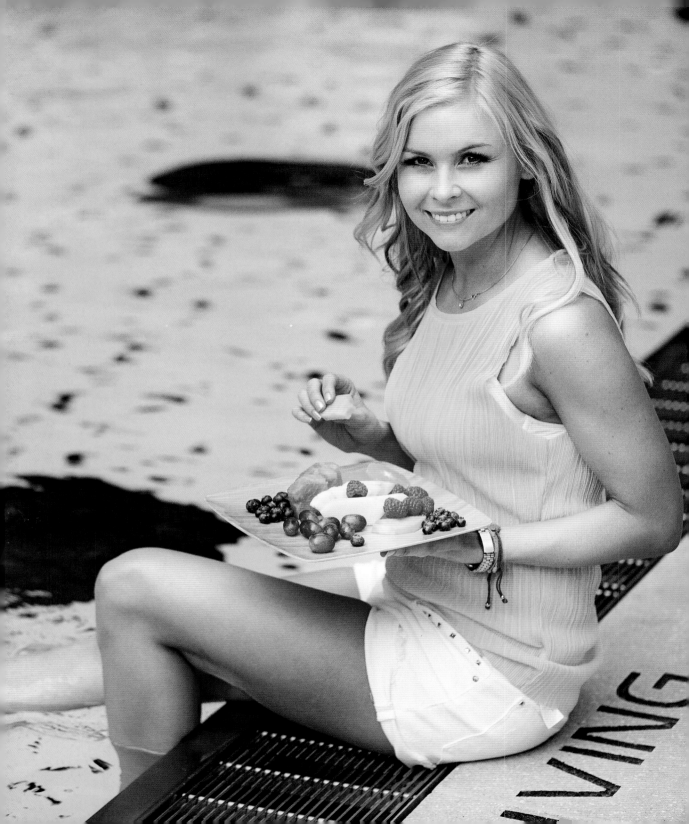

PART 2
NUTRITION

Julia Says

Perhaps I'm a new face for you? I've been in charge of the health pages in "Sofi's Mode" since a few years ago, and most recently, I've written as a health expert for "Aftonbladet Wellness" (the healthy living magazine published by a Swedish newspaper). But I haven't always been the person my girlfriends call up when they wonder what exactly hemp protein is useful for!

In the beginning of my career, I worked as a TV producer, a typical workaholic girl who combined twelve-hour workdays with late nights out. It was in the TV world that I met Sofi seven years ago. At that time, I was a segment producer on *Sofi's Mode*, and throughout the years, we've taken loads of trips together where, besides filming fashion weeks all over the world, we spiced up the program with fitness segments. We quickly noticed that these segments were at least as popular as the fashion segments.

After having worked for a few years in the hectic field of TV, where actually having time to eat lunch is a luxury, I finally felt that it was time to move on. I trained to become a nutritional advisor and began working full-time with what I think is the most fun of all.

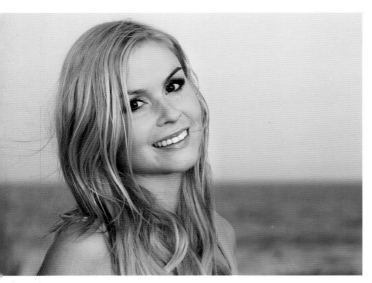

You might think that as a health journalist, you're guaranteed Gwyneth Paltrow's body and an interest in macrobiotic wheatgrass shots and Bikram hot yoga, yeah? Mm, well, that's not quite right. Like most others, I too have been a slave to daily coffee breaks with pastries. I also lost myself in the health jungle, testing everything from detox cures to LCHF without feeling that I ever found anything that really fit me and my lifestyle. Despite having a normal weight, I felt that just like many other girls, I was never properly satisfied with my body. I worked out regularly, but often treated myself to candy, sweets, and alcohol and then tried to compensate with more exercise, as atonement for my sins. The results were never there, and I was frustrated that nothing was happening.

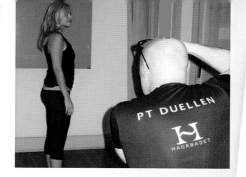

Before discovering a Bodylicious lifestyle . . .

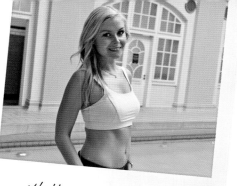

Hello, core muscles!

When I was going to get married last year, I wanted to get into the best shape of my life. I signed up for the "PT-duel," a competition at Hagabadet, a gym, spa, and restaurant in Gothenburg, Sweden, where you train with a personal trainer for ten weeks and get help to come up with a diet plan. When I went to weigh in, I was shocked! My weight was totally normal for my height, but my body fat percentage was 32. As a fit girl, you should be somewhere around 20 to 25 percent.

My personal trainer Sara Claesson, who has developed and quality-assured the Bodylicious fitness program, taught me how to train smarter and, above all, how to eat right to get results from my workouts. "Clean eating" is a common expression in the world of training.

I was sure I'd end up gaining weight, since I wasn't used to eating that much and that often, but the results were as clear as could be. Ten weeks later I actually weighed less, had dropped five inches from my waist, and had a body fat percentage of 24. I've continued to eat cleanly and work out three days a week, and today I'm in better shape than I ever dreamed possible.

Today, I've learned tons about clean, nutritious eating, and I know that it's absolutely the healthiest way to get in shape and stay in shape your whole life. It works whether your weight is normal and you just want a more toned, defined body, or you're overweight and need to lose some pounds.

I myself am a living example that it really works, and in this chapter, I'm going to share with you some of my best experiences and advice, supported by the latest research. If you follow them, I promise you that you'll feel better and be both happier and healthier.

Bodylicious, quite simply!

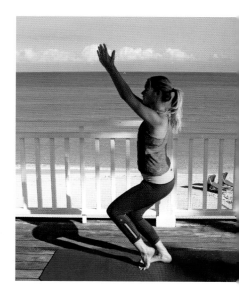

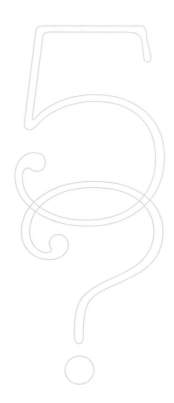

Julia's Five Most Common Questions from Readers

1. I live a healthy lifestyle and work out regularly but I don't get the results that I am looking for. What should I do to get my body in its best shape ever?

To overcome any training plateau, you have to surprise your body with some kind of new workout. Try interval training instead of plain running, and make sure to challenge yourself to go harder than you normally would—it should be difficult to talk at the same time. I personally use a pulse monitor, where I can clearly see how much I'm exerting myself. I often have a lot more to give.

Combine this with eating right, eating clean, and eating often—at least five times a day. Then you'll start seeing results.

2. What is your mind-set on those days you just want to scarf down a pizza and forget being productive?

I usually think about how I'm going to feel after I've eaten whatever I'm craving at the time. Is it worth feeling sluggish after a greasy pizza, or do I want to feel fresh and energized after a more healthy meal? That makes the choice easy. I also try to find better alternatives to the food I'm craving. For example, if I'm longing for chips, I might be just as satisfied with salty nuts. But if it's really pizza that I'm craving I will definitely have it. Eating by the 80/20 rule means no foods are ever banned.

3. I get off work at 7 p.m. and can't get to my workout before 7:30. I don't want to eat dinner before, but it gets so late, eating after. What should I do? I don't have the energy to exercise in the morning.

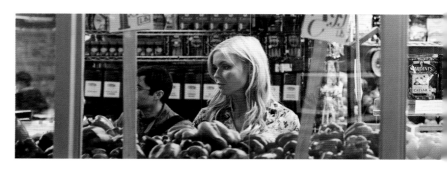

You need to eat both before and after your workouts to get the best results. If you exercise in the evening, I'd recommend eating a small meal at work, an hour or two before you train. Afterward, have a light dinner as soon as you get home, taking it easy with the carbohydrates. But for god's sake, don't skimp on the proteins.

4. I try to live a healthy lifestyle but my friends think I'm boring when I don't want to go out and party. What should I do?

When you start on a health journey, lots of people will get upset because they feel guilty about their own habits. Explain to them why your health is important for you and that you need their support. Who said you cannot go out and party without drinking? Have a non-alcoholic drink—nobody can tell the difference—and have fun with your friends. After a while, nobody will question you, and you can be 100 percent satisfied that you're sticking to your own health goals.

5. I work out about three days a week. Do I need protein powder or is buying a protein bar enough?

If you eat a balanced diet, protein powder isn't a must. Just make sure to eat something rich in protein after your workout so you can recover fully. If you have a stressful life, protein powder is a quick solution. I often have some myself after my workouts.

Skip the protein bars, though. Most of them are nothing more than disguised candy with a slightly higher protein content, and they contain as many calories and carbohydrates as a Snickers.

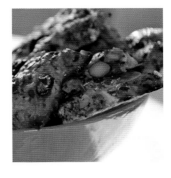

HOMEMADE PROTEIN BARS

2 egg whites

1 banana

1/2 cup (100 mL) protein powder

1 tsp vanilla powder (organic)

1/2 cup (100 mL) coconut flakes

1/2 cup (100 mL) chopped nuts

1/4 cup (50 mL) crushed linseed

1/4 cup (50 mL) sunflower and pumpkin seeds

1/4 cup (50 mL) dried cranberries or raisins

Mix all the ingredients into a smooth batter, pour onto a baking sheet, and bake at 340 degrees Fahrenheit (170 degrees Celsius) for eighteen minutes. Cut into perfectly sized pieces and store in the fridge.

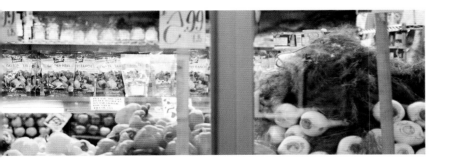

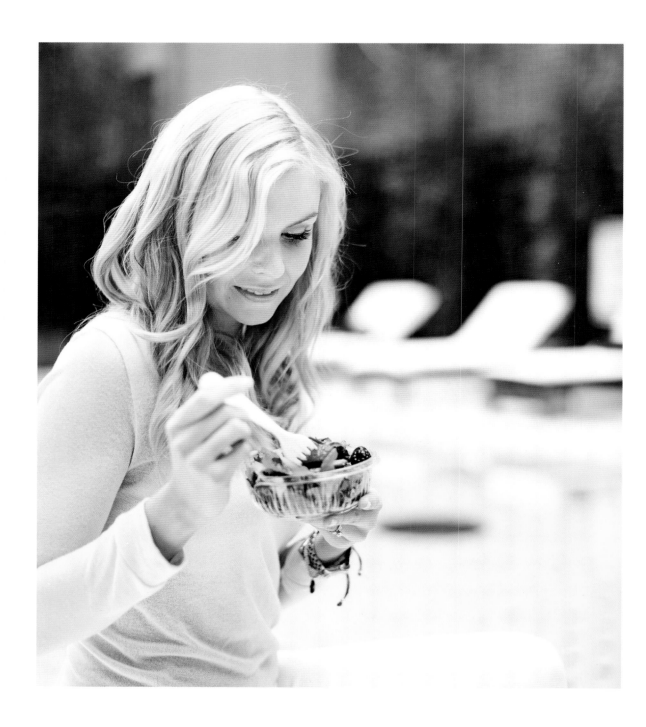

A Bodylicious Nutrition Plan

In the first section, you went through the fitness program with Sofi. But before you really begin your new healthy life, we want you to concentrate on one more thing: your nutrition, which I'm going to help you with now.

Why? Well, 70 percent of your results will come from what you put in your body. Yes, you read that right!

Unfortunately, it doesn't matter how much time and effort you spend on strength training, on the running track, or at the gym, if you're not eating right.

Learning to eat right will not only maximize the effects of your training and help you achieve results faster but it'll also turn your body into a fat-burning machine, which will make it easy for you to stay in great shape for the rest of your life. We're not saying you have to completely rebuild your life around some sort of complicated diet. We want to share with you our best tips for eating smart and finding a lifestyle you can stick to for an eternity. Yes, that means that wine, candy, and good food are all still allowed. But it also means that you'll have to learn to make smarter everyday food choices.

Eat the right food—not less food

Do you often think of Monday as your new life's starting gun, only to find that those healthy lunches are quickly replaced by drinks after work and take-out dinners in front of the TV?

Even if your goal is to eat healthfully, stress, deadlines at work, and dates—life, really!—can all put a spoke in the wheel when it comes to that healthy lifestyle you want so badly.

But there are tricks, and they won't require you to give up your after-work activities or never touch a single carbohydrate. There's no problem whatsoever with living an intense, fun life and still always feeling bikini-ready year-round. It's all about beginning to think smarter about food.

In this section, we'll go over how and what you should eat to give yourself the best foundation for shaping your body however you'd like it to be. We promise that you'll never have to feel hungry, feeble, or like you have to give up something. The secret to a toned body isn't low-calorie diets and working out like a maniac.

Eat often,
and enjoy it!
Eat more
and weigh less!

We've been bombarded with so many articles, commercials, and diets that promise quick weight loss that our attitudes about food have become skewed. Now we want you to forget all about those diets and focus on eating good, clean food. You don't need to count calories, either—when you eat the right food at the right time, it's not necessary. We want you to get energy from your food instead of losing it, and we want you to feel strong, healthy, and inspired to make good, healthy choices when you wake up in the morning.

One of the most common reasons we weigh too much or can't lose weight is that we quite simply eat too little. Yes, it's true! If you skip meals and cut back too much on the calories, your metabolism will drop down to an extremely low level of activity, and your body will put itself into starvation mode. Then, when you eat, your body will store everything you put into it, and you'll gain weight easily.

Do you skip breakfast and stave off your hunger with Diet Coke and a Starbucks latte? Stop that right now. The longer you keep on like that, the more you'll ruin your metabolism. What's more, all your workouts will be absolutely worthless if you don't eat properly. Another side effect of not eating regularly is that your body will release more of the stress hormones cortisol and ghrelin that break down muscle mass while encouraging the buildup of fat, especially around the stomach. If you choose the right foods instead, you can eat a lot, and still tone and sculpt your body. For the fat burning to kick in at the highest speed possible, it's quite simply of the utmost importance to eat substantially with clean, nutritious food.

Eat more often!

The faster your metabolism, the more calories your body burns every day. What affects your metabolism most of all is how often you eat and how much you move every day.

The first thing you should do to kick-start your metabolism is to make sure you eat often and regularly: five to six meals a day. Sure, that might sound like a lot, but this is the magic number that will program your body to a high-gear metabolism and perfect hormone balance. In addition to breakfast, lunch, and dinner, you should eat two smaller meals in between. These meals might feel unnecessary, but on the contrary, they're actually very important, partly because they keep your metabolism going, and partly because they stop you from snacking on other unhealthy things throughout the day. You'll find plenty of tips on what to include in these meals later (on page 136).

Don't skip meals! That causes your body to slow down its metabolism again. As a guideline, try to eat something every three hours. In the beginning it might feel like you're living on a timer, but after a while, you'll find that your body actually wants food this often—which is a sign that your metabolism is starting to get in gear.

Think 80/20!

Were you glued to Facebook all evening instead of going out and exercising? Did you eat a pizza on Tuesday night? Good god, nobody's perfect!

If you eat well 80 percent of the time, the remaining 20 percent won't play that big a role. Both Sofi and I live by this rule, which means cupcakes and evenings of Chardonnay are a natural part of our lives. Yay! We're no health robots, and eating cake on birthdays or having Mom's homemade potatoes au gratin for Sunday dinner is a part of life. By being able to allow ourselves some less healthy things now and then, we also get motivation to stick to good things the rest of the week. Let 80/20 be your mantra, and return to it whenever you're unsure about what you should eat.

And make sure you really enjoy it when you're going to eat something unhealthy. No more guilt! What's the point if you can't even enjoy what you just put in yourself?

Remember—it's what you do on most days that determines how you look and feel.

Carbohydrates build a tight body!

For many of us, everyday life without pizza, pasta, and bread is reality, and a sad one, at that! You might have learned to fear carbohydrates because you heard that they make you gain weight—but giving them up completely is not only incredibly dull and boring, it's also harmful to your body.

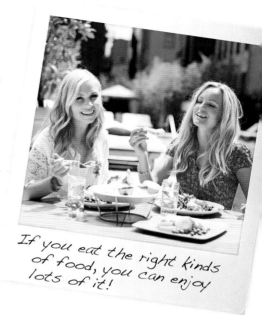

If you eat the right kinds of food, you can enjoy lots of it!

BODYLICIOUS *tip!*

Carbohydrates are the best fuel when you want to burn fat.

Carbohydrates are your body's favorite fuel, since they break down quicker than other nutrients: proteins and fats. If you're missing carbohydrates, you'll also be forced to decrease the intensity of your workouts, which in turn affects your results. Another nasty effect eliminating carbohydrates has on your body is that now, desperate for fuel, your body is forced to take fat from your liver and turn it into so-called ketones. Because your body prefers blood sugar in your brain, this ketone fuel is only 90 percent effective, which means you won't be on your mental A-game. If you're like us, living a hectic life where you juggle work, fitness, travel, family, and friends, it's simply not a smart solution.

Another side effect of consuming too few carbohydrates is that the serotonin levels in your brain plummet, which leaves many people irritated, depressed, and aggressive. We want you to wake up happy and full of energy!

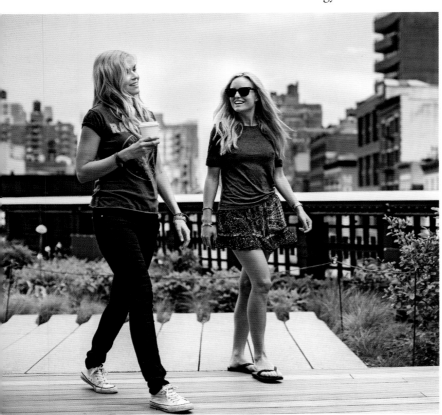

Choose slow carbohydrates like whole-grain bread and pasta, brown rice, quinoa, and vegetables, and you'll keep your blood sugar levels steady and decrease your cravings. Let about 30 to 40 percent of your daily food intake consist of good carbohydrates.

Refined carbohydrates, like instant pasta, instant mashed potatoes, and white bread, have been processed by machines that remove parts of the grain to give products a finer consistency and longer shelf life. In whole-grain products, all the parts of the grain are present (the hull, endosperm, and germ), along with important nutrients like B-vitamins, fiber, and iron. This also means that it takes longer for your body to break down these products, which means you get a lower glycemic index while feeling fuller.

bombs and make perfect natural flavorings for your yogurt, oatmeal, and desserts.

You should, however, eat somewhat less dried fruit. Because there's no water in them, the sugar concentration is higher.

Oh, how important water is

It's no coincidence that the most common accessory for models is a well-filled water bottle. If you don't drink enough water, 1½ to 2 liters a day, both your energy and weight will be affected. This might sound contradictory, but when your body doesn't get enough water, it actually stores more liquid, which causes you to become bloated and heavy.

Drink a big glass of water as soon as you wake up. Make it a habit to drink a glass with every meal. Keep a bottle with you in your bag wherever you go. And never forget to drink water before you exercise! People who drink lots of water also have faster metabolisms.

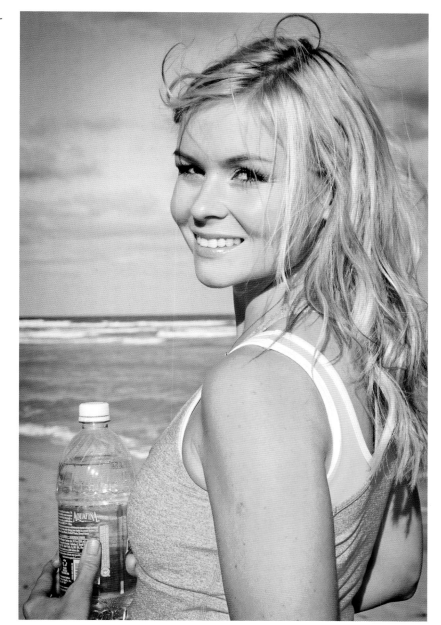

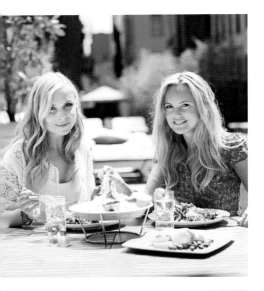

FOCUS ON WHOLE GRAINS,
EGGS, YOGURT, MILK, NUTS,
SEEDS, AND OTHER PROTEIN
SOURCES SO YOU STAY FULL ALL
DAY LONG.

Breakfast

You've heard it a thousand times: breakfast is the most important meal of the day. And the fact of the matter is that that's right. Even if you're stressed, tired, or simply not hungry, you shouldn't skip breakfast.

During the night hours, your body has been fasting, so it's important to eat something when you wake up to kick-start the burning of fat and calories. There are a number of studies showing that breakfast eaters tend to be thinner than those who don't eat breakfast, even though they consume more calories throughout the day. How does that work? Well, since your metabolism is kick-started in the morning, breakfast eaters are more active throughout the day and burn more fat and calories. What's more, your mental performance, in terms of memory, learning capacity, and problem solving are all boosted after eating breakfast because the carbohydrates give your brain fuel. If you're worried you just don't have time for breakfast, a slice of whole-grain bread with a layer of peanut butter or a yogurt with müsli or granola are my standbys. They take no more than a minute to make and you'll be consuming healthy fats and fiber that'll give you long-lasting energy and satiation.

Breakfast in the city

If you buy breakfast on the way to work, a plain yogurt cup with müsli, the Icelandic, protein-rich yogurt called *Skyr*, a cup of cottage cheese with nuts, and a banana or whole-grain roll with coffee are all good choices. Skip the drinkable yogurt, since it's nearly always filled with sugar. Granola bars and a lot of the other products you'll find on store shelves are out—even if they're described as being organic and rich in fiber. Most of these contain more sugar than a normal chocolate cake.

Will lattes make me fat?

Coffee itself contains no calories, but drinking at least 3/4 cup of regular whole milk a day can result in a gain of up to thirteen pounds in one year—pounds that sneak their way in and suddenly are just there. This isn't to say that you have to give up your daily latte, but try having it with skim milk instead, or enjoy a good old-fashioned smooth coffee with skim milk.

Love Juice

Nothing is as healthy and good for your body as fresh-squeezed juice or a smoothie with fruits, berries, or vegetables. Don't be fooled by packaging you see in stores with "fresh-squeezed" and "100% natural" slogans. All prepackaged juices and smoothies have to be pasteurized, which means that some of the nutrients end up being taken out.

On top of that, they often contain added sugar. The only way to get juice with the fullest nutritional value is to make it yourself or go to a juice bar. In the United States, it's easy to get your hands on freshly squeezed juices on nearly every street corner. Sofi usually buys her green juice at the gym around the corner. Unfortunately, these developments haven't come quite as far in Sweden, where there only are a select few health stores in big cities selling ridiculously expensive smoothies. Our solution? Make our own juice!

When you make your own juice, you don't need to peel the fruits, since much of the nutrient content is in the peel (but don't forget to wash the fruit thoroughly). The exception is citrus fruits, which you should peel so that the juice doesn't become bitter. If you find greens and vegetables boring, you can actually mix them in, too. You might, for example, upgrade your normal strawberry smoothie with a handful of baby spinach. The color will be a bit scary, but you won't actually get any of that "green" taste.

By replacing your after-dinner pastry with a fresh juice or smoothie, you'll eliminate your desire for sugary foods and instead start to crave healthy things. This is because juices contain high concentrations of nutrients and vitamins. A smoothie is also the perfect evening meal in front of the TV when you're hungry for something sweet.

Go crazy with coconut water!

SOFI: When I moved to New York three years ago, everybody was talking about this product called coconut water—news to me. In my juice bar, there were piles of green coconuts, and everybody was ordering different mixes with these coconuts. The first one I tried was with blueberries and banana, and I have to admit that it was love at first sip. Now coconut water is always in my refrigerator, and I like to have some after my workouts.

BODYLICIOUS *tip!*

Juicers are rather expensive, but they pay for themselves quickly since you don't have to keep buying prepared juices. Buy a new model with a built-in waste compartment so you don't have to clean it out manually, which is often a reason for these machines going unused. When you start using it, you'll quickly discover that the two minutes it takes to clean are well worth the trouble.

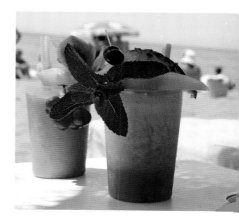

A super-drink we can't get enough of is coconut water. It's as good as Almond Joy and more hydrating than a sports drink.

If you haven't discovered coconut water yet, you have something to look forward to! Besides the exotic flavor that makes the perfect base for a smoothie, or just as a cool, refreshing drink, coconut water is a real health booster. It's free of artificial substances and naturally rich in calcium, phosphorus, sodium, potassium, zinc, selenium, iodine, sulphur, magnesium, bromine, and B-vitamins.

Because of its high nutritional value, it's considered better than sports drinks, which often have extra sugar added to them. Coconut water is recommended for anyone who isn't allergic to nuts.

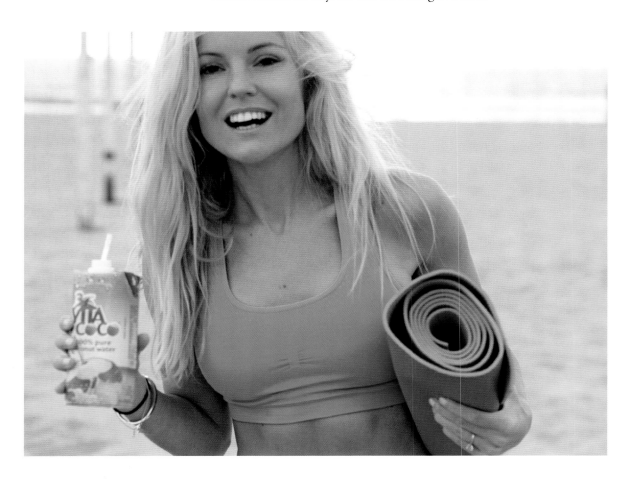

BEAUTY SMOOTHIE

- 2 apples
- 1 handful blueberries
- 1 handful raspberries
- ¾ cup (200 mL) light yogurt
- a few ice cubes
- a bit of cinnamon on top

This beauty-promoting smoothie is chock full of antioxidant-rich berries, which rejuvenate the skin and make it clear and smooth. A bit of cinnamon in the smoothie gives it extra warmth and spice.

DETOX JUICE

- 2 apples (golden delicious or royal gala)
- 1 carrot
- ¾ cucumber
- ¾ celery stalk
- 1 head of broccoli
- ½ red beetroot
- a few ice cubes
- 1 slice of lemon on top

This is the ultimate detox juice to kick-start your metabolism and give you an energy boost.

BACK ON TRACK SMOOTHIE

- 1 ¼ (300 mL) cups coconut water or plain water
- 1 large handful baby spinach leaves
- ¼ cup frozen mango pieces
- ½ banana
- a few ice cubes

Mix everything in the blender and top with ice. It'll help your body to recover, whether you've been out partying or you're suffering from jet lag.

BODYLICIOUS COCO-BERRY SMOOTHIE

- ¾ cup (200 mL) plain Greek yogurt
- ⅓ cup (100 mL) coconut water
- 1 ¼ cups (300 mL) frozen berries, like blueberries and raspberries
- 1 tbsp linseed oil
- 1–2 tbsp honey or agave syrup

Pour everything into the blender, drink, and enjoy!

Juices we love!

FLAT-TUMMY FOOD!

Have you heard the expression "core muscles are made in the kitchen"? It's true. You know those coveted six-packs? Let us tell you a little secret about those: you already have one! It's just covered by a layer of body fat, and if you want to make it visible, you've got to eat the right foods.

This is our top 7 list for foods that'll do your stomach some good and make it easier for your abs to come forward. Include them in your meals whenever you can.

1 YOGURT

Have you heard of probiotics? The probiotic bacteria—yes it's a bacteria that is actually good for you!—help to keep your digestive system in good working order. Yogurt is naturally full of these good guys that help your stomach work the way it should. The result: you'll naturally be rid of any bloating and have a flatter tummy. Plain natural greek yogurt is the healthiest choice.

2 ALMONDS

These delicious miracle snacks work wonders for your tummy. They contain a lovely cocktail of protein, fiber, vitamin E, and magnesium, which is important for building muscle tissue. Research has also shown that people who ate sixty almonds a day lost almost 50 percent more weight than those who ate the same amount of calories without almonds.

3 COLD-PRESSED COCONUT OIL

This oil literally serves as fuel for your metabolism. This is because its medium chain fatty acids are easier for the body to break down at the same time as they release heat and increase fat burning.

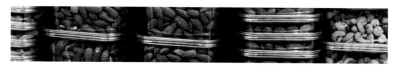

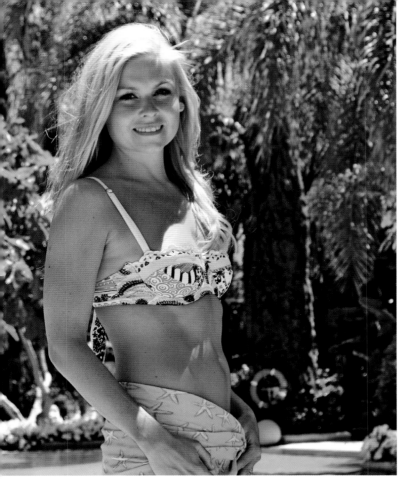

6 SALMON

The omega-3 fatty acids in salmon has proven to decrease inflammation and stress in the body. Salmon is also rich in vitamin D, which is important to a flat tummy. A lack of vitamin D makes it harder for fat cells to release and burn the fat stored in them.

7 WHOLE GRAINS

If you have a hard time getting rid of fat around your stomach, glycemic index–friendly carbohydrates like oatmeal are the solution. In a study, it was found that people who ate whole grains lost twice as much weight around their stomachs compared to those who did not. Whole grains minimize the production of insulin, which promotes the storage of fat.

4 BERRIES

Stress stimulates the production of the hormone cortisol, which tells your body to store more fat around your stomach. The antioxidants in blueberries and raspberries protect your body from stress and strengthen your immune system. They're perfect when it's time to give your tummy a sweaty workout.

5 ASPARAGUS

Asparagus contains the amino acid asparagine, which stimulates your body to break down fat. Asparagus is also a mild diuretic, so when you eat it, you'll quickly get rid of liquid if your stomach feels bloated.

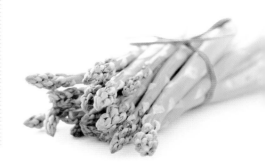

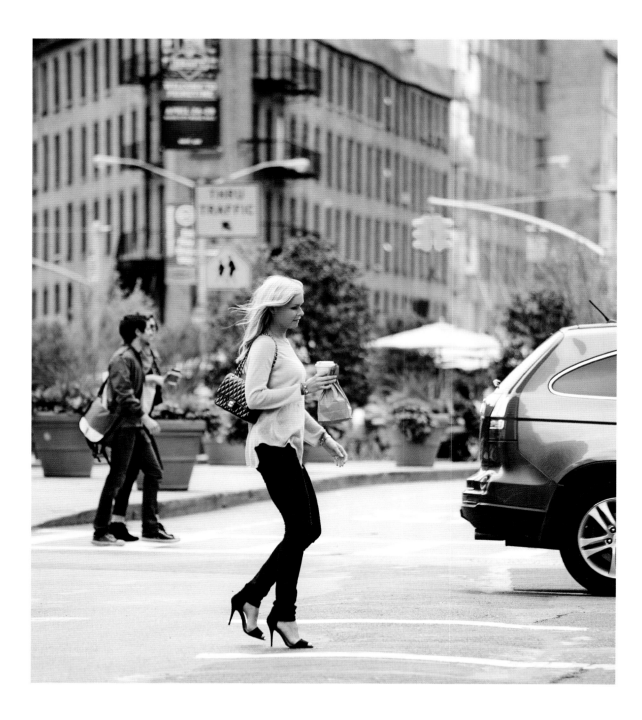

Lunch

If breakfast is the most important meal of the day, lunch is a close second. Here's where you should eat the biggest meal of the day, and really see to it that you're giving your body the right kind of energy for the rest of the day, especially if you're thinking about exercising after work or school.

Don't make a fuss about it. A wholesome salad is the ultimate lunch option. Make it with all kinds of different greens, some carbohydrate sources like bulgur wheat at the bottom, and chicken, tuna, shrimp, or salmon. Don't make the mistake of eating a protein-less salad, which can lead to cravings for sweets after an hour or two. Spruce up your salad with nuts, raisins, dried cranberries, sunflower seeds, and pumpkin seeds, and dress it with olive oil, lemon, and fresh spices. The possibilities are endless.

Super-lunch when you don't have the time

If you don't have time for lunch, a packed lunch is your best friend. It might sound boring, but you won't just save money—you'll get full control over the nutritional content of your food. This is one of the reasons that lunch boxes are common among, for example, fitness models.

The easiest way to start with a lunch box is to bring along the leftovers from yesterday's dinner. You can also take a few hours on Sunday to prepare some food for the coming week. I like to prepare a few steaks or chicken breasts and cook up a big batch of quinoa as the base of the week's salads. Then it only takes a few minutes to fix a tasty, healthful lunch. Invest in nice, fresh food storage boxes. Ones with built-in freezable blocks keep your food cool and fresh for up to seven hours.

Super-lunch at a restaurant

Lots of restaurants that serve lunch offer a daily special. Bodylicious-proof it by heading to the salad bar and filling an extra plate with greens and veggies. Try to make vegetables one-third of what you eat. Ask for sauces to be served on the side and try to choose whole-grain pasta, sweet potato, quinoa, or wild rice. Remember that restaurant portions are often much larger than the portions you make at home. If you feel full, ask for a box and eat the rest for dinner instead.

BODYLICIOUS *tip!*

Cook quinoa in vegetable broth for an extra-delicious flavor!

FOCUS ON VEGETABLES, BEANS, SALAD, SLOW CARBOHYDRATES, AND A PROTEIN SOURCE.

The snack attack!
How to outsmart your cravings

The snack attack—you know what we're talking about! It can strike without warning at any time, like when you're sitting at your desk and suddenly realize that you'd die for a pack of Swedish fish.

The best thing about eating according to Bodylicious principles is that it's fine to eat between meals. In fact, we recommend it! When you start eating regular small meals, your snack attacks will diminish and eventually disappear altogether. If you still have some mental cravings after that, we've got strategies to handle them.

Remember that snack attacks and cravings are not the same thing as hunger. Usually, some other basic need hasn't been met instead. Get to know your body's signals and what type of cravings you have so you can win the war against snack attacks.

Get to know your body's signals

Emotional cravings

Our cravings are often mental, and food is a quick, easy way to handle our emotions. If you're not feeling hunger from your stomach and ice cream is the only thing that can satisfy you, you can be certain you've got a mental craving on your hands.

To reduce typical emotional cravings, it's best to analyze what's triggering them. Has something happened in the last twenty-four hours or so that might have caused you to feel cravings? Perhaps you didn't sleep enough last night, missed a meal, or didn't eat enough for lunch? Make a list in your mind of possible options. Cravings usually don't last longer than ten minutes, so distract yourself by taking a walk or calling a friend.

Stress cravings

When you're stressed, it's easy to start gobbling down sweet, salty, and fatty junk foods. But junk food has a worsening effect—it raises your blood pressure and increases stress. So instead of slamming down a cheeseburger or a bag of chips when you've got exams or work on your mind, choose food that promotes the release of good, stress-reducing hormones in your body.

A slice of whole-grain bread with smoked salmon is an excellent stress meal. You'll get a natural boost of omega-3 fatty acids that make your brain produce more of the feel-good hormone serotonin. The whole-grain bread will give you a slow blood sugar curve that keeps your mood even and stable.

Fatigue cravings

There's a definite link between weight and sleep. The less you sleep, the more you eat. When you don't get enough sleep, your body's production of the hormone ghrelin increases, which sets off feelings of hunger, while levels of the appetite-suppressing hormone leptin are reduced. When you feel tired, it's also easy to reach for the fast carbohydrates that raise your blood sugar rapidly. Instead, go with slow carbohydrates like whole-grain pasta, brown bread, and müsli, which give you slow, steady energy, or take a short power nap, giving your body what it really needs.

PMS cravings

Does your body transform into an aggressive cookie monster the week before your menstrual cycle? It's not your imagination; right then, your estrogen and serotonin levels are especially low, and your body is longing for something to brighten it up. Vitamin B6 reduces the symptoms of PMS, so load up on B-vitamin-rich oatmeal and bananas for breakfast and chicken, turkey, or tuna for lunch and dinner. Good snacks include yogurt with pumpkin seeds, sunflower seeds, peanuts, and cashews; their high levels of magnesium will put you in a better mood.

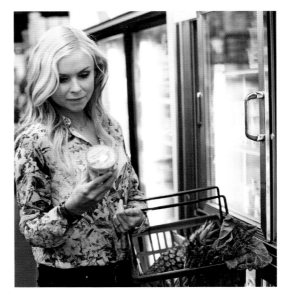

Sweet cravings

Are you always after something sweet? Erase sugar from your diet. The less sugar you eat, the less sugar you'll crave. Try reducing your carbohydrate intake and doubling your protein intake for a week. Proteins are the most filling nutrients, and when you feel full, your cravings for something sweet will let up. Chicken, turkey, cottage cheese, and soybeans are good choices.

Dinner

You started the day with a fierce kick-start breakfast, ate a power-lunch, and topped off with two small meals. All that's left now is the last meal of the day—dinner—and then you can be satisfied that your day has been completely bodylicious! For us, dinner is a social time, a perfect opportunity to socialize with family and friends. But for many, dinner is also that meal where good intentions unfortunately break down. If you've restrained yourself and "been good" all day, or if you've missed your smaller meals, there's a risk that you'll eat too much or choose poorly.

Dinner at home

If you cook at home, you have total control over what goes into your food. As a rule of thumb, always include protein, carbohydrates, and fats in your dinner; if you skip one of these, there's a greater chance that you won't feel full and satisfied, so you'll start craving something else. An easy trick to follow whether you're dining at home or eating out is that your protein source should be about the size of your open palm, your carbohydrates should be about half a cup, and you can fill the rest of your plate with as many greens and vegetables as you like.

Smart choices when eating out

So, cooking's not your strong suit? No problem! You can eat body-liciously even if you're eating out; Sofi does it all the time! As usual, keep in mind that you want to give your body food that's as nutritious as possible, and if there aren't any greens or veggies included in the dish you order, add on a side salad, or see if you can substitute a slow carbohydrate in place of a fast one. Not sure what to get? Pick the fish and fill up on vegetables; you'll never go wrong.

If bread baskets are like gold mines to you, choose the bread that contains the most whole seeds.

If you want to eat dessert, some sort of fruit salad, chocolate truffle, or sorbet with berries are some of the healthiest things you can choose from the dessert menu. And if that bombe or chocolate cake

Drink the wine and skip the bread!

FOCUS ON LEAFY GREENS, VEGETABLES, BEANS, LENTILS, AND PROTEINS LIKE FISH, CHICKEN, OR LEAN MEAT.

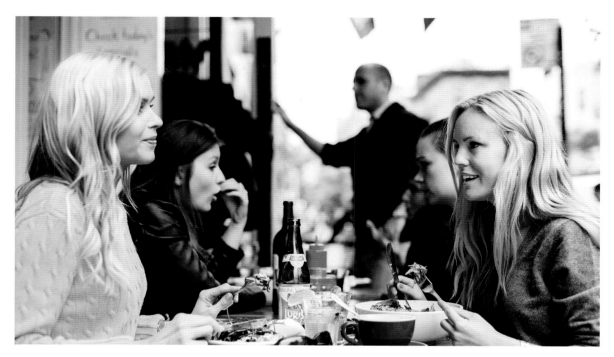

miraculously manages to appear on the table anyway, ask for two spoons and share it with your company. Sharing is caring!

Over the weekend and at parties

Weekends and parties can be difficult when you want to be healthy. You might sleep in, eat brunch, and go to a party or a movie when you're normally eating dinner.

The best way of tackling weekends is to stick to your routines. Try as best you can to eat normally, but skip a small meal if you sleep late in the morning, for example. If you're going to have a late dinner, it's best to have a small meal at the time you normally have dinner, so you don't risk getting super hungry and throwing yourself at the buffet as soon as you arrive at the party.

But also, don't forget to enjoy your treats! To live by the 80/20 principle means that you should regularly treat yourself without feeling guilt. Everything is OK to eat once in a while in reasonable amounts.

BODYLICIOUS tip!

Never skip a meal to eat sweets. Have that bag of candies after your food, so you'll be satisfied with less of it.

Here's How to Eat More Healthfully without Getting Bored!

Focus on good quality foods

Rule number one when it comes to food is to stop restricting yourself and to stop dieting. It is the worst thing you can do to your body because it's never sustainable and in the long run you'll just end up with a poor metabolism, less muscle mass, and a miserable mood. Instead, focus on eating five to six meals every day and treating your body to the most nutritious, clean foods, such as good fats, filling protein, and slow carbohydrates. When you choose good quality foods, you don't have to think about calories or restricting yourself.

Buy fresh products

Food that's been processed is full of additives, coloring, and preservatives that poison your body instead of providing healthy nutrients. Stop filling your shopping cart with these processed, ready-to-eat foods! When you start buying clean ingredients from the produce

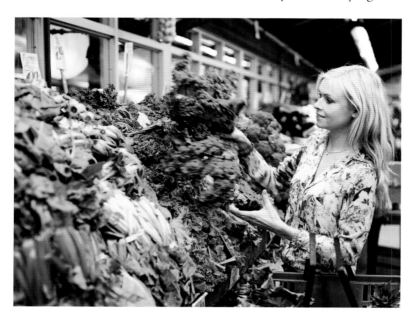

department and deli, you're already halfway to a healthier life. Remember—these are the departments where the fit girls get their food!

The one exception is protein powder, which is a good, quick solution for getting some protein in your body after a workout. But here, too, it's important to choose as good and clean a protein as you can. The Swedish company, Holistic, makes protein from whey produced by Swedish cows, without any sweeteners or artificial additives. You can buy it online or in health stores.

Learn to enjoy healthy foods

Why is it that you get those strong cravings for sweets, cookies, and candy? A likely reason is that when you were little, you had already eaten this sort of "reward food." You naturally want more of the things you eat regularly. But new research shows that you can weaken your old cravings and strengthen new, healthy ones by changing your eating habits. And it goes by quickly! In about five days, participants in the study who replaced their unhealthy snacks with healthful small meals craved these instead. The bottom line: eat better and healthier, and you'll naturally start longing for better, healthier food!

Add superfoods to your diet

A superfood is a food that's naturally rich in nutrients. By adding more of these superheroes to your daily foods, you'll naturally supercharge your diet. An easy tip for recognizing superfoods is color: the stronger and more vibrant the color (think blueberries, goji berries, spinach, and beetroots), the more nutritious the food is.

No diet food

Once and for all—you will not get slim from "diet products" like low-calorie shakes and "light" bars. Diet foods are the worst things you can eat since they're actually packed full of extra sugar and additives. If you want to lose weight, it's better to just eat a bit less of the full-fat, natural products. A typical diet shake often includes the equivalent of up to ten sugar cubes! What's more, the additives can make you bloated and leave you feeling hungry again.

Read the back of the package

If you only understand half of the ingredients on the back of the product, you can almost certainly find a better alternative. The problem when you eat too much of these fake ingredients is that they take up space from the nutritious food that you need to build up your natural immune system. A good rule of thumb to go by is that the more strange ingredients a product contains, the worse the quality probably is.

Stop dieting— eat cleanly instead

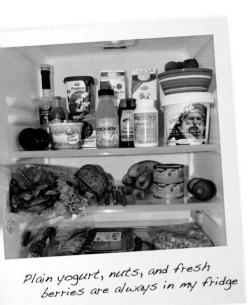

Plain yogurt, nuts, and fresh berries are always in my fridge

Be smart with your fridge

Can you guess what you usually take out of the fridge when you're hungry for something? Whatever's in front! The way your food is arranged at home plays an incredibly large role in determining how healthy your eating habits are. I try to always place healthy things like fruits, yogurt, and salad at the front of the center shelf, since I'll automatically eat more of them. Time to rearrange the fridge?

Replace salt with lemon

Too much salt in your food isn't just bad for your blood pressure; it also binds liquids in your body, which can make you bloated. One of the most common diet tricks in Hollywood is to completely eliminate salt one week before a big event. With a little fresh-squeezed lemon on your food, you'll instantly have more flavor without the unfortunate side effects of salt. Beware of pre-prepared food, too. Seventy-five percent of the salt we consume is already in the food we buy.

Plan

Time constraints are the most common excuse we women give for not eating better. Just like impulse shopping can lead to accidentally buying some random party top that just hangs there unused in your closet, impulse meals are the equivalent when it comes to food. If you don't have time, you've got to take that time elsewhere. Take advantage of weekends to set aside an hour or two to shop and prepare lunches and dinners for the week.

Don't be a perfectionist

Being too hard on yourself is a recipe for certain failure. After a few days of your insanely strict diet, it's easy to think "Oh, I ate a cookie, so I guess it won't make a difference if I eat the whole package since I already ruined my healthy diet."

Women who always say no to their favorite foods have higher levels of the fat-storing stress hormone cortisol, which means they'll have a harder time losing weight. If you want a cookie, go have one and enjoy it. But try to stick to just a few.

Decide to be consistent, not perfect

You can't eat perfectly every day, but you can be consistent. Eat better than you did before and try to achieve small goals. Then you'll see results.

Delicious morsels that aren't candy!

BANANA PANCAKES

We love to have these for breakfast, as a snack, or for dessert. You'd be hard pressed to find tastier, simpler sweet treats! They're so delicious that you really ought to have some right now, so why are you just sitting here reading this? Oh, right. You need the recipe.

    1 banana
    1 egg
    a few drops of vanilla extract
    1 pinch salt
    optionally, fresh fruit, berries, and
    agave syrup

Mash the banana. Beat in the egg, vanilla extract, and salt. Cook the batter in a frying pan. If you like, serve with fresh berries and agave syrup. If you'd rather make waffles, you can just as easily pour this batter into a waffle iron.

CHUNKY MONKEY

Do you love Ben & Jerry's "Chunky Monkey" ice cream? Then you've got to try our healthy Bodylicious take on it. This little ice cream is b-a-n-a-n-a-s! And it's perfect when you're hungry for something sweet.

    3 bananas
    ¼ cup (50 mL) chopped walnuts
    2 tbsp chopped dark chocolate

Peel and slice the bananas and place them in the freezer for at least an hour. Take them out and mix them with the walnuts and dark chocolate. Eat immediately.

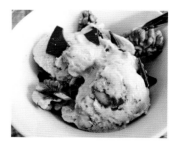

GINO WITH FRUIT AND BERRIES

This classic, fresh dessert often marks the end of our dinners. Enough for four portions.

    1 banana
    2 kiwi fruits
    1/3 cup (100 mL) blueberries
    1/3 cup (100 mL) raspberries
    7 oz (200 g) white chocolate
    1 tub mascarpone cheese
    Vanilla extract

Heat the oven to 350 degrees Fahrenheit (175 degrees Celsius). Peel and slice the banana and kiwi and place in a baking pan. Pour over the berries, shred or grate the white chocolate, and distribute it evenly over the fruit in the pan. Place in the oven for about ten minutes until the chocolate has melted. Add a few drops of vanilla extract to the mascarpone, and mix well to make a vanilla flavored cheese. Serve with a few spoons of the vanilla cheese.

LICORICE AND RASPBERRY ICE CREAM

Ice cream as preworkout fuel? You heard right! This protein-rich treat hits the spot! Licorice + raspberry = a combination that'll have your taste buds dancing the salsa.

    1 tub light cottage cheese
    1/3 cup (100 mL) raspberries
    2 tsp licorice powder (found in health food stores)

Mix the cottage cheese with the raspberries and licorice powder; put in the freezer for about thirty minutes before serving. Enjoy!

COCONUT AND CHOCOLATE MACAROONS

These are inspired by the raw food restaurant, One Lucky Duck, in New York.

    1 2/3 (400 mL) cups coconut flakes
    3 tbsp cocoa powder
    2 tbsp agave syrup
    4 tbsp coconut oil
    1/2 tsp vanilla extract
    1 pinch salt
    6 pitted dates

Mix all the ingredients except the dates in a bowl. Pit the dates and put them in a blender with the batter. Pulse until smooth. Roll into small balls and place on a plate in the fridge so they can firm up. Keep them refrigerated.

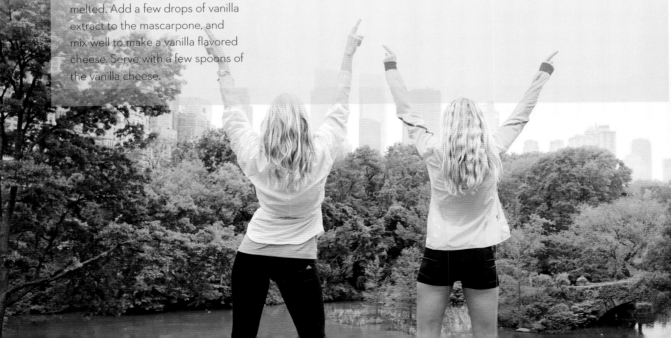

Fitness and Alcohol

A question we often get from readers is how we combine our fitness with evenings spent partying.

It might seem like an impossible combination, but you actually can live healthfully while still going to cocktail parties and red wine dinners. The secret is to judge when and how often it's worth it, what you're going to drink, and how you're going to help your body recover afterward.

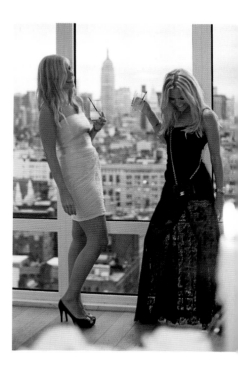

Make every other drink water

Alcohol has a negative effect on fat burning. Your body sees alcohol like a poison and focuses on breaking it down first. That means fat burning has to stop until all the alcohol's out of your blood. Drinking a lot of alcohol at once is also directly responsible for the breakdown of muscle tissue. Making every other drink a glass of water is a good rule.

So, how much is really OK to drink? A glass of wine won't ruin your workout, but after more than three drinks in one evening, you should take the next day off to rest. Never make the mistake of skipping dinner outright—then you'll only increase the risk of losing control later while also worsening your ability to resist poor choices. And yes, that pizza slice at 4:25 a.m. is one of them!

Working out the day after?

The biggest reason for feeling ill the day after is that your body is missing salts, minerals, and fluids. A light walk can be refreshing, but avoid intense exercise if you feel hungover. Post-drinking recovery puts a load on your body's organs. If you do intense exercise, you'll strain your body even more, and in the worst-case scenario, it can have a reverse effect, weakening your muscles and slowing your recovery. If you've had more than three drinks, it's better to just take a calm walk and let your body rest.

Working out and partying the same day?

You should avoid intense exercise immediately followed by going out and partying like crazy, since you won't get any benefit from your workout then. Besides that, if you've been sweating a lot before a night out partying, your liquid levels are already in the red, and you can look forward to a deluxe hangover the next day. If you work out the same day you're going to a party, try to schedule your workout earlier in the day, so you don't go straight from the gym to the pub. Pouring alcohol into your body right after a workout will drastically lengthen your recovery time. For this reason alone, it's especially important for you to consume restorative carbohydrates and protein after your workout, before uncorking anything.

Reset button?

Skip the Bloody Mary and other "restorative" drinks and go with water instead, or why not coconut water? It's extra good, since it's rich in electrolytes. We also like fluid replacement drinks like Resorb. It generally takes around two hours for your body to break down a glass of wine, and a full twenty-four hours for your body to restore the balance after a night of drinking.

Don't forget to eat regularly, either. The day after those drinks, your blood sugar plummets, making you crave sweets while also causing you to feel tired and out of sorts. The trick here is to avoid lying down on the sofa with a capricciosa. Eat your five meals as normal, don't skip any meals, and drink extra water. Let wine and other drinks be a bonus for those days when they're worth it, but never look on them as excuses to skip your workouts or eat unhealthy food.

Sipping skinny?

A glass of red is the "healthiest" choice you can make if you're going to drink alcohol. In addition to it's numerous positive effects—preventing cardiovascular disease, fighting against poor circulation, among other things—red wine boosts your body's fat burning. Cabernet Sauvignon has especially high levels of resveratrol.

White wine and champagne?

Choose as dry a wine as possible, since dry wines contain the least sugar. If you compare wine and champagne, there's often more sugar in the champagne, which makes the wine a better choice in terms of glycemic index. On the other hand, champagne glasses are typically smaller than wine glasses.

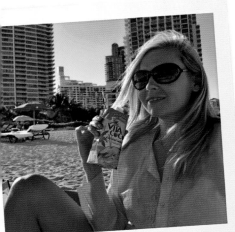

Don't forget to hydrate your body the day after.

Which drink options do we go for?

Strong spirits generally don't contain any carbohydrates at all, though they do contain more calories. A good rule when trying to choose as small a drink as possible is to go for clear alcohol. Choose vodka or gin before whiskey, bourbon, and rum. Avoid all drinks containing cream or milk ingredients, as well as sugary drinks and hard drinks. The sugar in these drinks not only adds calories but can make your hangover drastically worse.

Examples of low-calorie drinks include vodka lime soda and so-called "spritzers," which are half wine and half soda.

GOOD CHOICES	
1 glass red wine	110 calories
1 glass white wine	100 calories
1 spritzer, with white wine and sparkling water	85 calories
1 glass champagne	90 calories depending on sweetness. Prosecco contains 60 calories per 100 mL, but Moët & Chandon contains 83 calories in the same amount.
1 vodka soda	64 calories
1 gin and tonic	150 calories
1 skinny margarita	about 96 calories

OK ONCE IN A WHILE	
1 strong beer	190 calories. Try to choose bottled beer instead of beer on tap. Bartenders will pour larger drinks when serving beer on tap.
1 Cosmopolitan	150 calories. As many calories as a soft-serve ice cream.

THE WORST OFFENDERS	
1 piña colada	644 calories and 20 g of fat
1 frozen strawberry margarita	720 calories, as the drink is often served in big two-cup glasses.
1 mojito	242 calories, almost as much as a cinnamon bun! Ask the bartender to tone down the sugar and use more lime and sparkling water.

Figures are approximate. Calorie content varies with the size of the glass and other factors.

SKINNY MARGARITA

Pour ½ fl. oz tequila, the juice of one lime, and a splash of cointreau or triple sec. Mix with lots of ice to obtain a smooth, flowing margarita. Dampen the rim of a martini glass with a wedge of lime and dip in a mixture of half salt and half sugar. Pour in the drink. Did somebody say "cheers"?

Smart tips for when you've sinned!

Oops!

Oops! I drank the bar dry yesterday . . .

We'll admit it, even we do that sometimes. Let go of that hangover anxiety; hopefully it was worth it!

What you need to do now is restore the balance of fluids in your body, and food is what's most important here. Just because you sinned yesterday doesn't mean you can crush today too, with the "I was hungover" excuse.

We usually drink a vitamin-rich juice instead of Coca-Cola and eat a tasty cheese omelette instead of pizza. Forcing more unhealthy food on yourself the day after will only make things worse. Try tossing a little asparagus into that omelette; it contains an enzyme that breaks down the alcohol more rapidly.

Oops! I thought I was smoking hot with a cigarette!

The fact that our discretion worsens in the course of a night spent partying is no secret. The result is a cough, hoarse voice, and an especially nasty hangover. Look around you. How many people who were smoking five years ago still smoke today? Who today doesn't know how dangerous smoking is? And how uncool it is? It's really time to replace those little white sticks with something else. A kiss, a cool sorbet, or the knowledge that tomorrow morning will be cough-free. Take along a friend with the same problem and reward yourselves the day after when you successfully abstain from cigarettes for an entire evening.

Oops! I didn't make it to my workout this week, either . . .

Some weeks are like fashion week in New York, where the only cardio you get is running like a madwoman from tent to tent in four-inch heels. Look on the bright side: a week off of your training isn't going to destroy what shape you're in now. If you exercise a lot, it can even be a good idea to take a week to rest and let your body fully recover. Does one week quickly turn into two or three? Get out your calendar and plan your workouts as if they were as important as meetings with your boss. Think of this, too: right now, people who are even busier than you are working out.

Oops! I had a trans fat party!

Sometimes, your body is just screaming for the absolute worst kind of fat—if you've tried truffle fries, you know just what we're talking about!

Don't be too hard on yourself. It's obviously not a good idea to stuff yourself with trans fats every day, but once in a while is not the end of the world. Just make sure that your next five meals are of the good kind. What you eat most often is what builds up your body.

Oops! I went bananas at Magnolia Bakery.

Go with a proper, protein-rich breakfast the day after your cake- or candy-based revelry; an omelette is a good choice. Then continue eating something rich in protein every three hours, which will stabilize your blood sugar again. Also avoid fast carbohydrates and sweet drinks like juice, smoothies, and frappuccinos. Why not take advantage of those spring-loaded glycogen reserves and go for a sweaty spinning workout or a run? You'll appreciate the extra kick of energy!

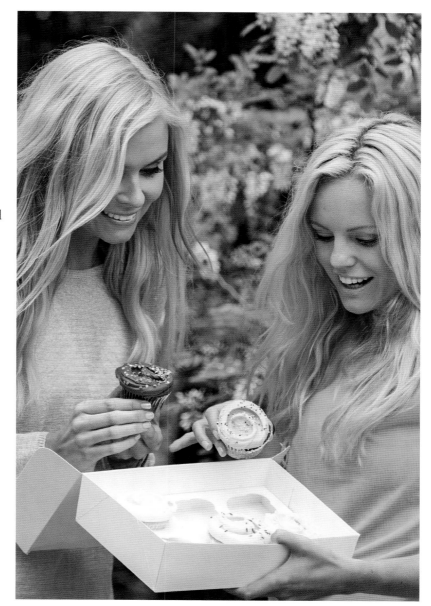

10 FAT-BURNING SNACKS

As you know by now, snacks are your secret weapon to increasing your metabolism. When you eat something smaller in between larger meals, your body understands that more energy is on its way, preventing it from producing more fat-storing cortisol and slowing down your metabolism. Choosing the right snacks can even give your metabolism an extra turbo-boost. Here are our 10 favorites.

1 SALAD WRAP

Make a healthy wrap by replacing the tortilla with a large leafy green. Fill with tuna salad, meat sauce, or a fresh tomato salsa.

2 APPLE & PEANUT BUTTER

The fiber in the apple reduces cravings for sweets, in addition to containing pectin, which limits the amount of fat that can be absorbed by your cells. With a tablespoon of unsweetened peanut butter, you'll be consuming healthy fatty acids and filling protein.

3 HARD-BOILED EGG

Boil some eggs and keep them in the fridge so you always have a snack when hunger starts to set in.

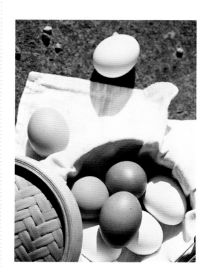

4 CINNAMON COTTAGE CHEESE WITH APPLE

Cottage cheese is both low in fat and high in calcium, which has a positive effect on fat burning. Sprinkle some cinnamon on top and you'll also drop your body's insulin levels, which inhibit the burning of fat if they're too high.

5 PROTEIN PANCAKE

By adding a scoop of protein powder to your batter, you can easily turn pancakes into fat-burning snacks. Since the protein takes more energy than carbohydrates and fats to break down, you'll increase your fat burning while staying full longer.

6 WHOLE GRAINS & FRESH CHEESES

Fiber is the easiest way to stop fat from lodging itself in your body. It keeps your digestive system in good order and makes you feel full.

7 AVOCADO & SUNFLOWER SEEDS

Avocados are full of healthy monounsaturated fatty acids. A substance called L-carnitine can also be found hiding in the creamy fruit. It's commonly added to weight loss products because it increases the production of energy in muscle cells.

8 COTTAGE CHEESE WITH BERRIES

Berries mixed with light cottage cheese are a match made in heaven. Raspberries are especially good for fat-burning because they contain a type of ketone that increases the burning of fat.

9 GREEK YOGURT

Greek yogurt with chopped walnuts, a tablespoon of linseed, and a sliced banana is one of the simplest snacks you can throw together. Try to choose Greek yogurt with more protein than normal in it. Nuts and linseed give you healthy fatty acids.

10 SMOKED SALMON ON TOAST

Spread fresh cheese on a slice of whole-grain bread and top it with salmon. Salmon is packed full of healthy omega-3 fatty acids.

Montauk

St. Moritz

Fitness on Vacation

Working out regularly and eating right while traveling is a challenge for many. But there are tricks.

SOFI: I hardly even notice anything strange anymore. Traveling is a part of my life. To me, flying is like taking the bus. The distance between Stockholm and New York feels smaller than any flight within Europe. For me, it's about not distinguishing travel days from normal days. I love routines, and I have a tendency to make patterns so that all I have to do later is press play. Time to catch a flight: play! Here are my tips:

1.   I always try to have a sleep deficit before I get on a plane. The best time in the world to sleep is when you're on a plane. I've often dozed off before the wheels even leave the ground. I love flying! Nobody can get ahold of me, I don't need to answer emails, and I can relax for the better part of awhile. Airlines that offer in-flight Wi-Fi really aren't my thing. I leave my phone and laptop in my carry-on, which I store above my seat, never to be seen until we've landed.

2.   I don't eat airplane food. I make sure to have a proper meal before I get to the gate. I fill up as I normally would and make sure to actually feel full. Then I just stock up on water and nuts.

3.   When I land, there are three things on my mind: Resorb, a moisturizing facial mask, and a run. Always. Swollen calves and adjusting to the time zone require an extra go. Since I sleep through the flight, I always have energy to head out for a nice, calm run with good music in my ears.

4.   No matter if I'm at work, at home, or on vacation, my diet looks more or less the same. New York has taught me to love healthy, yet delicious, alternatives. Avocado, egg, excellent

sushi, juice bars, and frozen yogurt on every street corner. Of course, there's plenty of ice cream in my vacations, but not every day. Remember my and Julia's 80/20 strategy!

5. On vacation, I like to follow the customs of wherever I travel. In Mexico, I order fish tacos and guacamole; in the Alps, cheese; and in southern France, olives and shellfish. Try to find the best wherever you are.

JULIA: Don't destroy your good results just because you're on vacation. Here are my three best tips to stay healthy even while traveling.

1. On the ground—The air pressure is such that all the food has to be heavily salted to even taste like anything. Add empty carbohydrates and you'll get that bloated stomach directly. When I have time, I make it to the airport well in advance so I can buy something there to take on board. A favorite in Sweden is Naked Juicebar in Arlanda, which has fresh salads, wraps, smoothies, and energy bowls. Even a twelve-piece sushi meal is a better choice than some airlines' definition of "dinner": a cheeseburger and a bag of potato chips . . .

2. In the air—I always buy an extra water bottle after checking in. That's a must, since the dry air in the airplane dries me out. Even if the flight might be more fun with wine, it's worth sticking to water until you land, fresh and ready for your vacation!

3. Once you're there—If there's one time you want to feel especially sexy, it's when you're on vacation. I think that's motivation enough to make healthy choices. I usually think like this: I can enjoy everything, but not all at once! When you're away for a week, you can't eat all the goodies in one day; spread them out! Then you'll have plenty of time to taste your way through the delis.

BODYLICIOUS *tip!*

Kick off your shoes and enjoy a run along the beach. Since it's more challenging for your feet to fend off the movable sand, more muscles are engaged, and you get a more effective run.

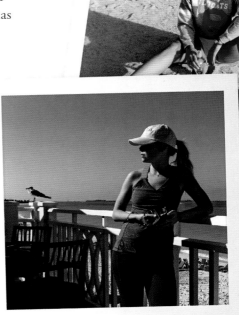

Miami and the Bahamas

A day—my food diary

13 APRIL, 5:11 PM / FOOD AND DRINK / WRITTEN BY SOFI

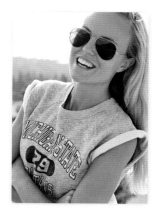

Good morning: I feel like the most clichéd model writing this, but I always start my morning with a ton of water. Two or three glasses.

Breakfast: Right now, I'm in the middle of a blueberry kick. Greek yogurt, a handful of blueberries, honey, and chopped walnuts. Then I drop by the juice spot in my house and order a "green juice with pineapple." I'm pretty bad about eating greens in general, but with this green liquid in my body, I feel like Popeye.

Before noon: Grabbing a *caffè latte* at my favorite place in Chelsea Market (9th Street Espresso). Drinking it in the taxi on the way to a meeting. Since I only drink one of these a day (I get way too jittery otherwise and can't sleep), I don't bother with the "skinny lattes" and have one with regular milk.

Lunch: My favorite lunch is Eggs Florentine (especially from Café Cluny in the West Village). I love eggs! Particularly like this, with greens, salmon, and hollandaise sauce.

Snack: I always want something sweet in the afternoon. When I moved here, it was easy to just swing by Magnolia Bakery, but that got to be unsustainable, so now I've found a healthier alternative: frozen yogurt from Pinkberry!

Author, moderator-editor, and TV hostess.

CATEGORIES:

general,
clothes,
shoes,
food and drink,
beauty,
health,
personal.

BLOG ARCHIVE:

April,
March,
February,
January,
. . . older posts

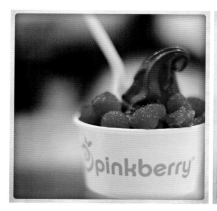
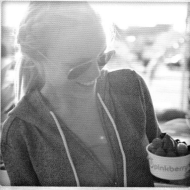

Dinner: Grilled corn and fish tacos. I'm sitting here working at my computer, so it'll be an order from La Esquina. Thanks for all the delivery food, New York! I have to admit though, there's not a whole lot of homemade food in this city. Ordering food to your home generally costs about the same anyway.

Film snack: Watching a film with my fiancé. When I moved here, I was tipped off to the existence of One Lucky Duck, and they've got some absolutely lovely little treats that aren't even that unhealthy. Munching on some coconut and chocolate macaroons with a cup of chamomile tea.

That's all for today!

A day—my food diary

22 APRIL, 8:42 A.M. / WRITTEN BY JULIA

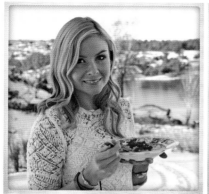 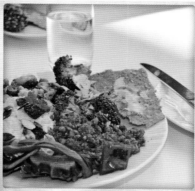

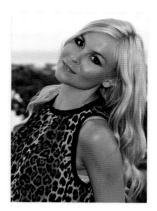

nutritionist, beauty and
health journalist.

CATEGORIES:

diet,

playlist,

news, personal,

recipes,

beauty,

Sofis mode,

fitness.

BLOG ARCHIVE:

April,

March,

February,

January,

. . . older posts

Breakfast: I like to start with something warm, like grits. I also feel a lot fuller compared to if I ate yogurt. I mix it up by adding berries, banana, apple, or nuts and cinnamon.

Snack: Cottage cheese with blueberries and walnuts is a favorite I almost always have at home in the fridge. Takes only two minutes to fix.

Lunch: Salmon is my all-time favorite food. I eat it any way I can. Grilled, cured, smoked, as sashimi or tartare. You can't go wrong with a crisp salad on the side.

Snack: If I'm in a hurry, usually a smoothie from Blueberry or Naked Juicebar. I'm in love with Blueberry's "Eat Your Greens Shake." If I'm at home, an apple with cinnamon and cottage cheese.

After working out: Protein shakes. I usually just use water, but if I want to make a luxury shake, I use about a cup of soy milk, the same amount of coconut water, a scoop of protein powder, two handfuls of baby spinach, some chunks of frozen mango, half a chopped banana, and then I blend all that with ice.

Dinner: Hamburger patties, fish, or chicken with bulgur or brown rice and a big, wholesome salad to go with it.

Dessert: I love making raw food treats with a bit of stuff I already have at home. Nuts, dates, cocoa powder, coconut oil, and coconut flakes can become yummy balls to keep in the fridge and take out in the evening.

As you can see, it's quite possible to eat deliciously yet cleanly. Focus on protein, carbohydrates, healthy fats, and flavor your food with cinnamon, berries, fresh herbs, and lemon; you won't even miss those nutrient-less quick energy meals.

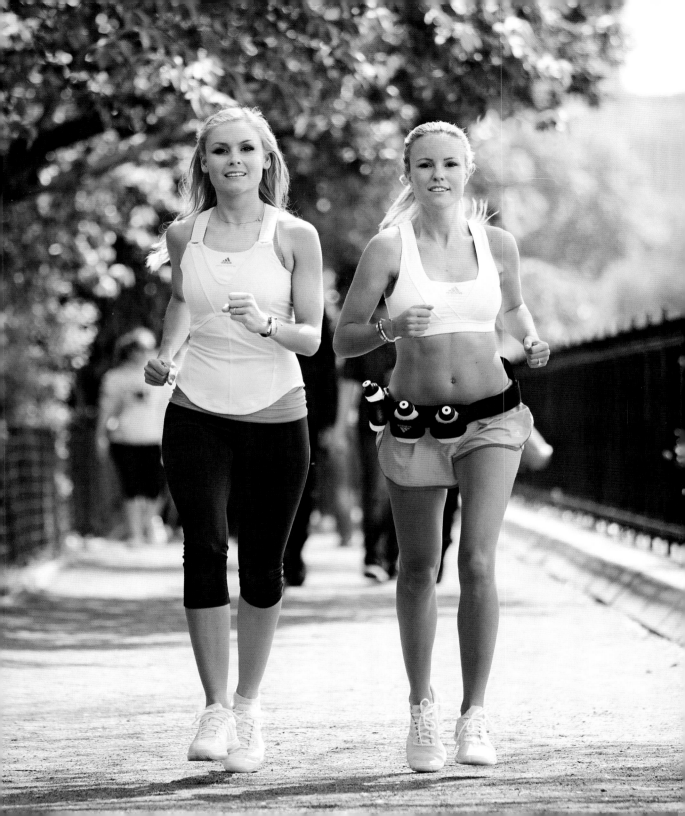

PART 3
BIKINI
BOOT CAMP

3-week Bikini Boot Camp

Are you ready to get started and sculpt your dream body?

Twenty-one days is all the time you need to make changes to your life that'll really stick. After those three weeks, your new lifestyle will have become a habit, and cravings for old bad habits will have disappeared.

Having a clear goal is good for your motivation, so why not plan something festive for the end of the program. Also prepare yourself to feel so good and love your results so much that you won't want to stop after twenty-one days!

Get ready for three exciting, challenging weeks where your body will be sculpted to no less than your very best self. If you can dream it, you can make it real!

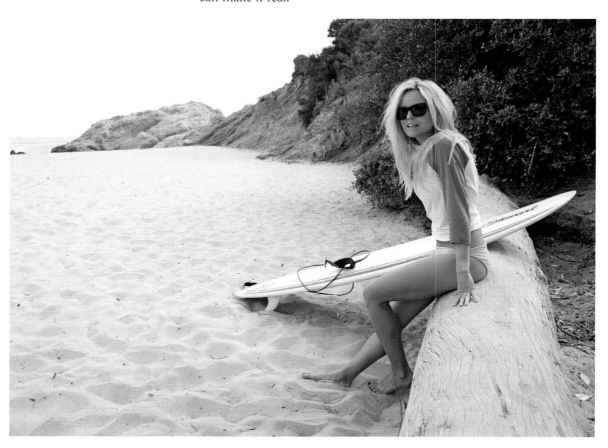

WEEK 1							
	MONDAY	**TUESDAY**	**WEDNESDAY**	**THURSDAY**	**FRIDAY**	**SATURDAY**	**SUNDAY**
Morning	30-minute walk before breakfast	Rest	30-minute walk before breakfast	Rest	30-minute walk before breakfast	30-minute walk before breakfast	Rest
Afternoon/ evening	Booty and core	Rest	Legs and arms/shoulders	Rest	Back/chest and core	Bikini-Fit	Rest

The importance of rest

You build muscles not when you're working out but when you're resting. When you exercise, microscopic tears occur in the muscle fibers. When you rest, these tears are repaired, strengthening the muscle mass. That's why it's important that the muscle group you just worked out gets a chance to repair itself for at least forty-eight hours before you work it again.

Good breakfasts:

- Plain yogurt with berries and müsli, a heavy sandwich, and an egg
- An omelette with two eggs, a splash of milk, baby spinach, and sliced turkey, with a heavy sandwich on the side
- Oatmeal: ½ cup of high-fiber oats, 1 tbsp linseed, 1 tbsp sunflower seeds, 1 tbsp pumpkin seeds, 1 cup water, berries or banana, a pinch of salt, and milk

Good lunches:

- Chicken breast, fish, lean beef, or turkey with quinoa, brown rice, bulgur, wheat berries, Khorasan wheat, or spelt; as much salad, vegetables, or veggie stir-fries as you like

- Whole-grain wrap with brown rice, greens, and chicken, shrimp, or tuna
- Salmon or chicken over a wholesome salad with bulgur and lots of vegetables; dressing made with olive oil, fresh herbs, lemon juice, and balsamic vinegar

Good dinners:

- A grilled steak, hamburger patties with sun-dried tomatoes and feta cheese
- Fish in the oven or chicken with as many vegetables as you like; ½ cup of a carbohydrate source like quinoa, wheat berries, bulgur, or brown rice

Sauces:

- Try using cottage cheese or ricotta as a base
- Homemade hummus or tzatziki is perfect with meat and fish

Small meals:

- At least two per day!
- Treat yourself! Enjoy our sweet treats on pages 129–130 about once a week

WEEK 2							
	MONDAY	**TUESDAY**	**WEDNESDAY**	**THURSDAY**	**FRIDAY**	**SATURDAY**	**SUNDAY**
Morning	30-minute walk before breakfast	Rest	30-minute walk before breakfast	30-minute walk before breakfast	30-minute walk before breakfast	30-minute walk before breakfast	Rest
Afternoon/ evening	booty and core	Rest	Legs and arms/shoulders	Rest	Back/chest and core	Interval training	Rest

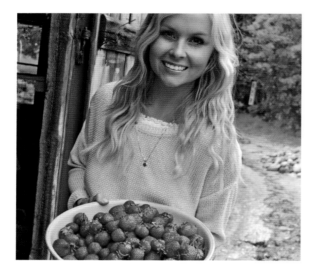

BEAUTY *tip!*

The quickest way to achieve a nice glow is the bronzing creams Per-fékt and Body-Bling, developed by Jennifer Lopez's makeup artist Scott Barnes. We use them on our legs and décolletage.

Nutrition, week 2

By now, you've probably started noticing the advantages of eating clean and nutritious food. Don't forget that when you eat is at least as important as what you eat. Give your body something to work with every three hours and you'll keep your metabolism on top! Take this day guide as an example of what a good food day can be, and adapt these approximate times to work with your everyday schedule:

- Breakfast: after your morning walk (around 7:30 a.m.)
- Snack 1: two to three hours after breakfast (around 10:00 a.m.)
- Lunch: two hours later (around 12:30 p.m.)
- Snack 2: three hours later (around 3:30 p.m.)
- Dinner: three hours later (around 7:00 p.m.)
- Optional evening meal: at least two hours before going to bed

WEEK 3							
	MONDAY	**TUESDAY**	**WEDNESDAY**	**THURSDAY**	**FRIDAY**	**SATURDAY**	**SUNDAY**
Morning	30-minute walk before breakfast	30-minute walk before breakfast	30-minute walk before breakfast	30-minute walk before breakfast	30-minute walk before breakfast	30-minute walk before breakfast	Rest
Afternoon/evening	Booty and core	Rest	Legs and arms/shoulders	Rest	Back/chest and core	Interval training	Rest

Nutrition, week 3

You've bought the dress, and now it's hanging at the very front of your closet. The last thing you need a week before your big event is to feel bloated and swollen. Even if you've eaten a healthy diet for the last two weeks, there are some foods, even the healthy ones, that can cause bloating. A good rule of thumb is to cut down on these for the final week leading up to your event:

- Vegetables like broccoli, cauliflower, onions, and beans, which should form a part of your healthy diet, can create bloating when they're digested in the stomach. If you know you have a sensitive stomach, keep these to a minimum for the last few days before your event. Eat them cooked instead of raw.

- Sweeteners like aspartame, sucralose, xylitol, and sorbitol (found in sugar-free chewing gum and diet sodas, among other things) are hard for your body to break down and can cause your stomach to swell.

- Alcohol can make your body bloated and puffy—your face, too. You know, that hungover look that isn't particularly flattering on anyone…

Fitness

Sara Claesson is a personal trainer and nutritionist, dancer, and dance instructor. She's put together the fitness program on the following pages using the exercises Sofi shows us in the exercise section. Each workout is designed to bring your heart rate to the max, increasing your overall fat- and calorie-burning.

Where you see, for example, "twelve reps," you should repeat the exercise twelve times in a row without stopping. When you see, for example, "x3," this means you should rest about thirty seconds after those twelve reps, perform twelve more, rest thirty more seconds, and perform twelve more. That, then, would make for a total of thirty-six reps.

BEAUTY *tip!*

Eyelash extensions are a beauty trick that we love. You'll always look lively and avoid having to apply makeup there for a few weeks. Bling Lash in New York is Sofi's favorite.

BOOTY AND CORE

Sumo kick (good for warming up) 24 reps, p.36
Reverse lunge kick, 24 reps, p.38

x 3

Maximum heart rate

Squat with jump, 12 reps, p.35
(Keep a fast, steady pace; this should be tough)
Mountain climber, 12 reps per leg, p.45

x 3

Split squat, 24 reps, p.39
Toe plié lunge, 12 reps, p.37
Booty press, 24 reps, p.40
Scissors, 25 reps, p.46
Plank, 30 seconds, p.47
Side plank, 40 seconds, p.48
Heels to the skies, 25 reps, p.49
Full jackknife sit-ups, 12 reps, p.50

Perform all these exercises as in the description. Rest briefly between exercises and repeat the entire routine a second time, if you want an extra-hard workout.

LEGS AND ARMS/SHOULDERS

Squat with lift, 30 reps, p.25
Shoulder press, 12 reps, p.60

x 3

Maximum pulse rate

Side lunge with hop, 12 per side, p.26
Burpees, 12 reps, p.76

x 3

Single leg squat, 6 per side, p.27
Squat with star, 24 reps, p.28

x 3

Curtsy lunge, 12 reps, p.29
Shoulder fly, 12 reps, p.58
x 3 (can be combined into one exercise)

Upward-facing booty press, 24 reps, p.30
Plank with dumbbell rows, 12 reps, p.59
T push-up, 6 reps, p.61
Side triceps push-up, 24 reps, p.62

Perform all these exercises as in the description. Rest briefly between exercises and repeat the entire routine a second time, if you want an extra-hard workout.

SARA'S PERSONAL TRAINER *tip!*

If you already work out regularly and are used to exercising, you can add Bikini-fit interval training or running intervals on one of the rest days.

BACK/CHEST AND CORE

Weight boxing with scissor jump, 2 minutes, p.67
Flat-back fly, 15 reps, p.68
Diagonals, 24 reps, p.69
Push-up with leg raise, 12 reps, p.71
Superwoman, 12 reps, p.70
Y-T-I, 12 reps, p.72
Mountain climber, 12 reps, p.45
Scissors, 25 reps, p.46
Plank, 30 seconds, p.47
Side plank, 40 seconds, p.48
Heels to the skies, 25 reps, p.49
Full jackknife sit-ups, 12 reps, p.50

Perform all these exercises as in the description. Rest briefly between exercises and repeat the entire routine a second time, if you want an extra-hard workout.

BIKINI-FIT

Burpees, p. 76	10–12 reps
Sumo kick, p. 36	12 reps per side
Explosive lunge jump, p.78	20 reps x2
Mountain climber, p.45	15 reps
Triceps dips, p.80	6 reps per side
T push-ups, p.61	10–15 reps

Perform all the exercises one after another in sequence.

BIKINI-FIT INTERVAL TRAINING

Tabata intervals have been called the world's most effective training. It's been shown that four minutes of high-intensity Tabata intervals have a better effect than a whole hour of low-intensity training.

You'll need a clock or phone with a timer/stopwatch, along with paper and pen. If you have a smartphone, you can download a Tabata app.

Start with the Bikini-Fit exercises, performing the first exercise as many times as you can in 20 seconds. Now rest for 10 seconds.

During the break, write down how many repetitions of that exercise you managed to do. Repeat eight times before moving on to the next exercise.

So for each exercise, your workout is as follows:
8 x 20 seconds intense work
+ 8 x 10 seconds rest
= 4 minutes

The entire workout will take 24 minutes.

SARA'S PERSONAL TRAINER *tip!*

Turn your workout into a competition against yourself and try to manage more and more repetitions in each set. Always try to beat the number you did last time, even if it's only by one repetition!

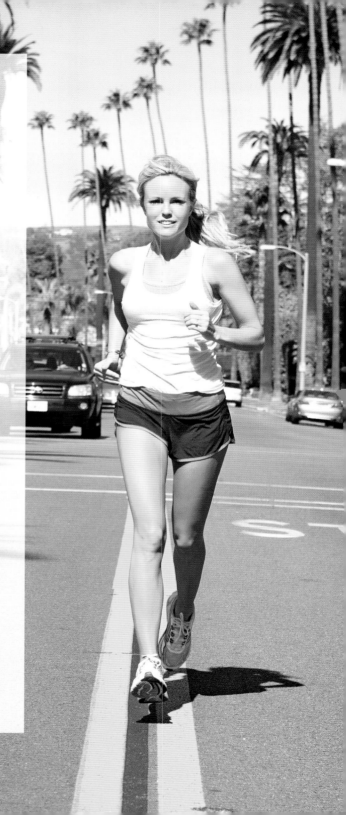

BODYLICIOUS RUNNING INTERVALS

Interval training where you alternate between running at top speed and taking a short recovery is ultra-tough. But it's also one of the most effective things you can do if you want to burn fat and tone up your body rapidly. Just like Tabata intervals, you'll burn just as much fat and achieve the same health benefits with short, intense workouts as with longer medium-intensity workouts.

2+3 minute intervals

You can do this set at a running track or anywhere outside your house.

Start by running at a moderate warm-up pace for 5 minutes. Continue at a fast run for 3 minutes. This should be around an 8 or 9 out of 10 on your personal toughness scale.

Recover for 2 minutes.

Max out for 3 minutes.

Recover for 2 minutes.

Max out for 3 minutes.

Recover for 2 minutes.

Max out for 3 minutes.

Recover for 2 minutes.

SARA'S PERSONAL TRAINER *tip!*

Since most songs are around 3 minutes long, you can easily create an interval training playlist with songs that get you pumped. Choose 6–8 songs, half of them shorter and calmer, the other half longer, more upbeat songs. Select your playlist and alternate running quickly and calmly in time with your music. The time will absolutely fly!

7-day Bikini Boot Camp

By now, you know we're not about unrealistic diets and quick fixes. But sometimes you want to give your normal routine an extra kick. That's why we created this 7-day Bikini Boot Camp. It's not a lifestyle, but an intense week for whenever you want to give yourself a real health kick. One example of a time we both did this real pulse-quickener was the week before we shot the cover of this book. Julia gave it her all and followed it to the letter before her wedding, and she looked and felt simply smashing! It's an intense week, but if you follow it, we guarantee you'll both feel and see the results!

NOTE: This program is for fully healthy people over the age of 18. If you're unsure before beginning a diet and fitness program, you should always ask a doctor for advice.

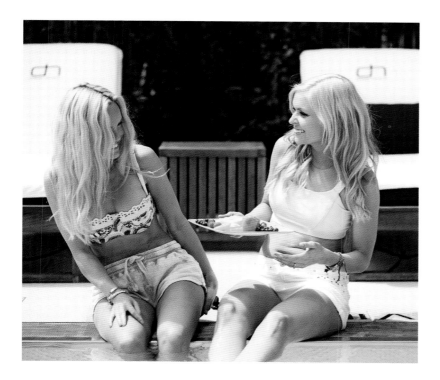

BODYLICIOUS *tip!*

Stay away from soft drinks, alcohol, and fatty or salty meals, which put the brakes on your stomach and bowels, preventing them from burning fat and calories optimally. Focus on regularly eating food that's as clean as possible.

NUTRITION PROGRAM

DAY 1

Morning walk: 30–45 minutes. Drink a big glass of water and perhaps a cup of coffee first.

Breakfast: Oatmeal with ½ cup mixed blueberries and raspberries, cinnamon, and milk. One hard- or soft-boiled egg.

Snack: A sliced apple with ½ cup cottage cheese, some halved walnuts, and cinnamon.

Lunch: Grilled salmon fillet with ½ cup quinoa or wild rice, a big salad, and mixed greens with our Bodylicious dressing: ½ cup balsamic vinegar, 2 tbsp olive oil, juice of 1 freshly squeezed lemon, juice of 1 freshly squeezed lime, 1 tsp sea salt, and 1 tsp dijon mustard.

Snack: Omelette with two eggs, a bit of milk, baby spinach, and chopped turkey slices.

Workout: Booty and Core (see pp. 34, 44).

Dinner: Oven-roasted chicken with herb cottage cheese, grilled broccoli, and a big, wholesome salad.

DAY 2

Morning walk: Same routine as day 1.

Breakfast: 1 ¼ cups light yogurt with ½ cup unsweetened müsli, 1 chopped fruit, a large sandwich with turkey and paprika.

Snack: 10–15 unsalted plain almonds.

Lunch: Whole-grain wrap with chicken, brown rice, beans, and greens.

Snack: 1 handful unsalted plain almonds and a fruit.

Workout: Bikini-Fit (see pp. 75, 149).

Dinner: Pork tenderloin with tomato salsa; mixed greens with avocado, asparagus, beans, lentils, and sunflower seeds.

DAY 3

Morning walk: Same routine as day 1.

Breakfast: Omelette made with two egg whites and one egg yolk, a splash of milk, 3 chopped turkey slices, 1 handful baby spinach, ⅓ cup (100 mL) chopped tomatoes, 1 tbsp pumpkin seeds.

Snack: 1 sliced apple with a tablespoon of plain, unsweetened peanut butter.

Lunch: Whole-grain wrap with cottage cheese, avocado slices, smoked turkey, and a wholesome salad.

Snack: Shape-up smoothie (recipe, p.95).

Workout: Legs and Arms/Shoulders (see pp. 24, 56).

Dinner: Oven-grilled salmon fillet with lemon, mixed greens, and edamame.

DAY 4

Morning walk: Same routine as day 1.

Breakfast: 1 ¼ cups (300 mL) plain yogurt with ⅓ cup (100 mL) müsli and fruit salad; 1 hard- or soft-boiled egg.

Snack: Two slices of smoked salmon on a slice of whole-wheat bread.

Lunch: Lemon chicken with a quinoa salad and cottage cheese with herbs.

Snack: ½ avocado with roasted sunflower seeds.

Workout: Bikini-Fit (see pp. 75, 149).

Dinner: Beef patties with sun-dried tomatoes, feta cheese, and olives with greens, olive oil, and balsamic vinegar.

DAY 5

Morning walk: Same routine as day 1.

Breakfast: 1 ¼ cup (300 mL) light yogurt with ⅓ cup (100 mL) müsli and chopped fruit. A big sandwich with turkey and paprika.

Snack: 1 hard-boiled egg with ⅓ cup (100 mL) peeled shrimp.

Lunch: Lamb meatballs with bulgur and vegetables.

Snack: Light cottage cheese with blueberries and some walnut halves.

Workout: Back/Chest and Core (see pp. 66, 44)

Dinner: A steak or oven-grilled fish with lemon and chili. Tomato salsa and a wholesome salad with Bodylicious dressing (see day 1).

DAY 6

Morning walk: Same routine as day 1.

Breakfast: High-fiber oatmeal with ⅓ cup (100 mL) mixed blueberries and raspberries, cinnamon, and milk. 1 hard- or soft-boiled egg.

Snack: 7 fl oz (200 mL) plain yogurt with ¼ cup (50 mL) raspberries and some walnut halves.

Lunch: Shrimp or tuna salad with egg, mixed vegetables, and quinoa.

Snack: Carrot sticks with hummus dip.

Workout: Bikini-Fit (see pp. 75, 149).

Dinner: Stir-fry with vegetables and chicken breast. Mixed greens with avocado, asparagus, tomatoes, beans, lentils, and sunflower seeds.

DAY 7

Morning walk: Same routine as day 1.

Breakfast: High-fiber oatmeal with ⅓ cup (100 mL) mixed blueberries and raspberries, cinnamon, and milk. 1 hard- or soft-boiled egg.

Snack: 1 handful almonds and some fresh pineapple slices.

Lunch: Baked salmon with coriander and lime sauce (fresh coriander, lime juice, and crème frâiche or sour cream), vegetables, quinoa, ½ avocado.

Snack: Shape-up smoothie (recipe, p.95)

Workout: 30 minutes of jogging or 20 minutes of running intervals.

Dinner: Oven-grilled cod, salmon, or haddock fillet with lemon, chili, and lightly browned asparagus. Big salad and tomato salsa.

DAY D

Don't make the mistake of cutting down on food right before your event. Fasting before a party is the worst thing you can do. First, you risk being so hungry that you get drunk off the first glass of champagne; second, you risk eating too much of the food served at the event and ending up bloated.

Stick with your normal five meals throughout the day, with protein and slow carbohydrates that give you a long-lasting, stable feeling of being full. Eat a snack before heading to the event and don't forget to enjoy how fantastically sexy, healthy, and fresh you are. Treat yourself to something you really love—you're worth it!

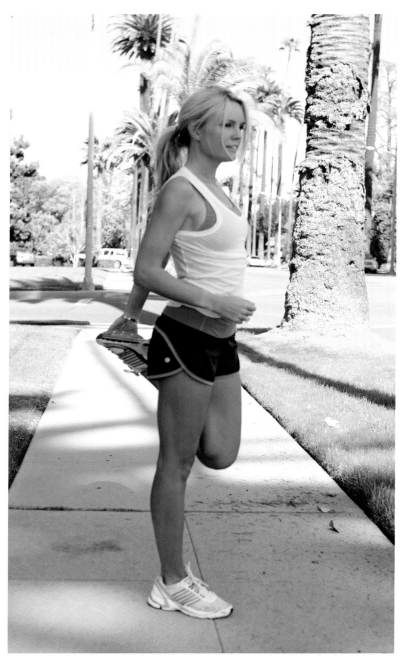

How much should I eat?

We don't think you should count calories, since it's not necessary when you eat cleanly and regularly. There's a difference between how calories from different foods affect your body. Three hundred calories from chicken will affect your body differently than three hundred calories from candy, as protein contains all the nutrition you need and requires more energy from your body to burn.

To more easily know about how much you should eat, to give yourself the the right amount for your build, use your hands as a guideline. As a guideline per meal, ready-made carbohydrates should fit in your cupped hand. The protein source should fit on your open palm. You can generally eat as many vegetables and leafy greens as you'd like.

Also set a goal to eat until you're just full enough, before you go into a food coma. Listen to your body, eat a little slower, and enjoy the flavors.

10 REASONS TO LOVE YOUR BODY

1 Nobody is like you; your body, smile, and personality make you completely unique. Nobody else can ever copy it.

2 Even if you're not always good to it, your body stands by you every day and always gives you another chance. It's never too late to upgrade your life.

3 It's lovely to be a woman: we have intuition, the capacity to multitask, and we're always one step ahead of the guys in sex appeal. Enjoy your womanliness and sexy feeling.

4 Your body sends you warning signals when something's wrong. The two of us have both felt signals warning us of stress and poor health habits. How cool is it to know that you have your own personal alarm bell? Listen to your body; it's fantastic.

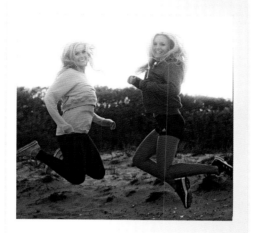

Bodylicious!

5 Working out and eating right are investments in the future. No, we'll admit it, when we were twenty we might not have thought that way. But now, when we look around, it's clear which women are setting good and bad examples. A healthy life can beat any La Prairie cream.

6 Don't be so hard on yourself. Not everything is about how your body looks. A smile, a sparkle in your eyes, self-confidence, and self-esteem are at least as

sexy as a well-sculpted bum. Just ask any guy.

7 When you treat your body well, it shows. When we were writing this fitness book and thinking a little extra about how we ate and worked out, we saw instant results. If you reward your body, it'll reward you back.

8 Think of all the fun you and your body have together! You can climb, dance, have sex, run at Mission Impossible speeds, and do cartwheels!

9 Even if you are your own worst critic, there's someone who absolutely adores your body type.

10 Love your body—now. You'll regret not having done so when you're older. Who hasn't looked at old pictures and wondered why they weren't more satisfied back then?

Bikini Boost!

Our final tip: think like a Brazilian! There's nothing sexier than someone who wears a bikini with self-confidence—regardless of the body inside it. In Rio, you'll see more skin than fabric, tiny triangle bikinis that hardly leave anything to the imagination but exude sexiness. We Swedes are too restrained sometimes; dare to show off your curves! And promise you'll try your way through a bunch of different bikinis to see what fits you the best. Don't settle for the same old stuff. It's easy to get the idea that you fit one particular style and that one alone. In *Sofi's Mode*, we always push for daring to try new things. Break away from old ways and help yourself!

Take a look around the next time you're at the beach or the next time you spend a day out in the city, for that matter. What catches your eye? We're certain it won't be that magazine-perfect body, but the one that radiates "I love my body." We hope that this book has inspired you to live more healthfully and to give your body a boost with fitness and energy. Now it's up to you to soak up all our tips. Good luck!

XOXO
Sofi & Julia

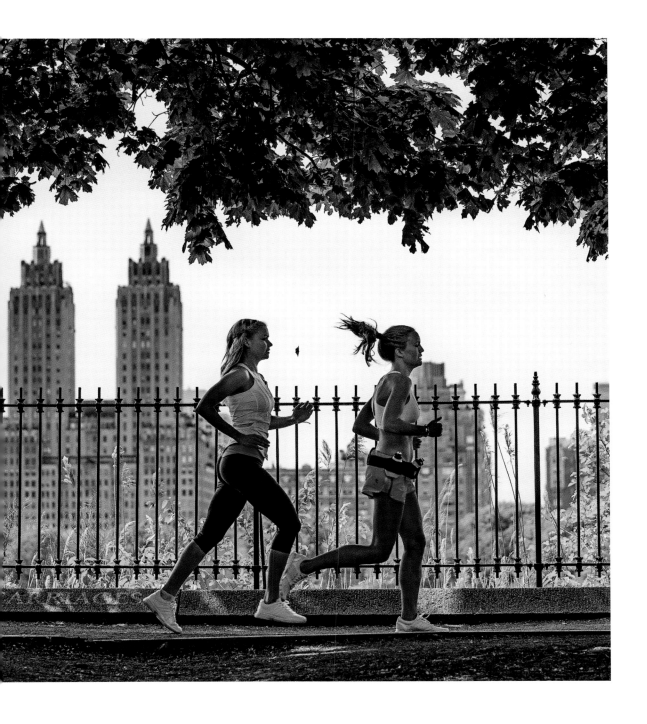

References

P. 19: *High-intensity interval training is time efficient and effective, study suggests.*
Wiley, Blackwell. ScienceDaily 2010.

P. 83: *Regulatory accessibility and social influences on state self-control.*
vanDellen, Hoyle. Personality and Social Psychology Bulletin. Department of Psychology, University of Georgia 2010.

P. 93: *Timing protein intake increases energy expenditure 24 h after resistance training.*
Hackney, Bruenger, Lemmer. Department of Kinesiology, Michigan State University 2010.

P. 94: *Caffeine Improves Physical and Cognitive Performance during Exhaustive Exercise.*
Hogervorst, Bandelow, Schmitt, Jentjens, Oliveira, Allgrove, Carter, Gleeson. Sports & Exercise 2008.

P. 109: *Dietary Protein and Exercise Have Additive Effects on Body Composition during Weight Loss in Adult Women.*
Layman, Evans, Baum et al. The Journal of Nutrition 2005.

P. 110: *Natural responses to visual food stimuli after a normal vs. higher protein breakfast in breakfast skipping teens.*
Leidy, Lepping, Savage et al. University of Kansas Medical Center and University of Missouri 2011.

P. 114: *Skipping breakfast can lead to unhealthy habits all day long.*
Institute of Food Technologists (IFT). ScienceDaily 2012.

P. 118: *Almonds vs. complex carbohydrates in a weight reduction program.*
Wien. Journal of Obesity. City of Hope National Medical Center, California 2004.

Green Tea Catechin Consumption Enhances Exercise-Induced Abdominal Fat Loss in Overweight and Obese Adults.
Maki, Reeves, Farmer, Yasunaga et al. The American Institute of Nutrition 2009.

P. 119: *The effects of a whole grain–enriched hypocaloric diet on cardiovascular disease risk factors in men and women with metabolic syndrome 1 2 3.*
Katcher, Legro, Kunselman et al. Pennsylvania State University 2008.

P. 127: *Health halo effect: Don't judge a food by its organic label.*
Wan-Chen Lee, Wansink Cornell. ScienceDaily. Federation of American Societies for Experimental Biology 2011.
Dietary monotony and food cravings in young and elderly adults.
Levin-Pelchat, Schaefer. Monell Chemical Senses Center 1999.

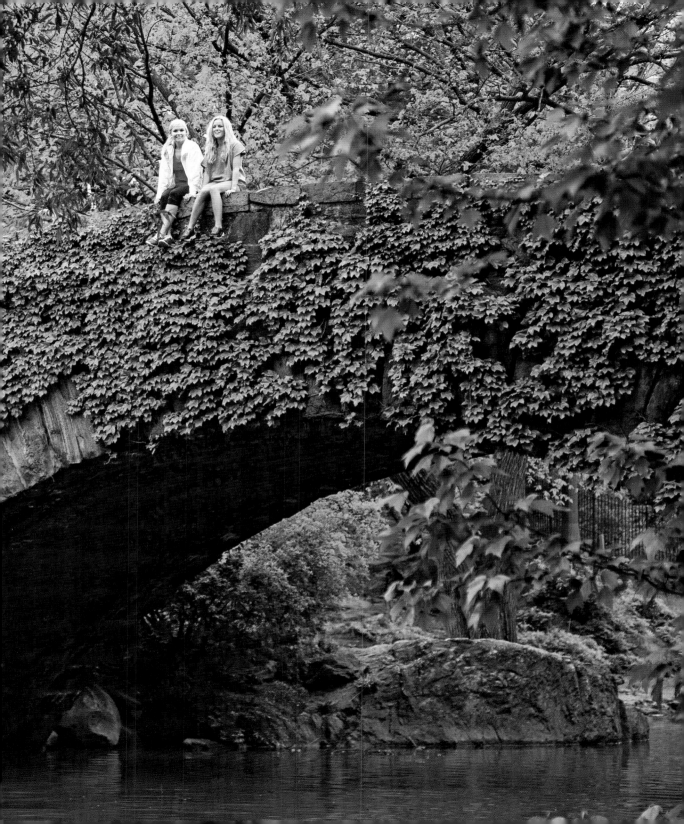

INDEX